Pi Gu Chi Kung

Pi Gu Chi Kung

Inner Alchemy Energy Fasting

Mantak Chia and
Christine Harkness-Giles

Destiny Books
Rochester, Vermont • Toronto, Canada

Destiny Books
One Park Street
Rochester, Vermont 05767
www.DestinyBooks.com

Destiny Books is a division of Inner Traditions International

Library of Congress Cataloging-in-Publication Data
Names: Chia, Mantak, 1944- | Harkness-Giles, Christine.
Title: Pi gu chi kung : inner alchemy energy fasting / Mantak Chia and
    Christine Harkness-Giles.
Other titles: Inner alchemy energy fasting
Description: Rochester, Vermont : Destiny Books, [2016] | Includes
    bibliographical references and index.
Identifiers: LCCN 2015038183| ISBN 9781620554258 (pbk.) |
    ISBN 9781620554265 (e-book)
Subjects: LCSH: Fasting—Health aspects. | Detoxification (Health)
Classification: LCC RA784.5 .C455 2016 | DDC 613.2—dc23
LC record available at http://lccn.loc.gov/2015038183

Printed and bound in the United States by Versa Press, Inc.

10 9 8 7 6 5 4 3 2 1

Text design by Priscilla Baker and layout by Virginia Scott Bowman
This book was typeset in Garamond Premier Pro with Present and Diotima used as
    display typefaces

Photographs by Sopitnapa Promnon

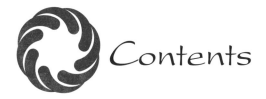

Contents

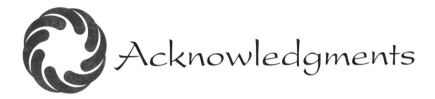# Acknowledgments

The authors and Universal Healing Tao Publications staff involved in the preparation and production of *Pi Gu Chi Kung: Inner Alchemy Energy Fasting* extend our gratitude to the many generations of Taoist masters who have passed on their special lineage, in the form of an unbroken oral transmission, over thousands of years. We thank Taoist Master Yi Eng (One Cloud Hermit) for his openness in transmitting the formulas of Taoist Inner Alchemy.

We offer our eternal gratitude to our parents and teachers for their many gifts to us. Remembering them brings joy and satisfaction to our continued efforts in presenting the Universal Healing Tao system. As always, their contribution has been crucial in presenting the concepts and techniques of the Universal Healing Tao.

We wish to thank the thousands of unknown men and women of the Taoist healing arts who developed many of the methods and ideas presented in this book. For their continuous personal encouragement, we wish to thank our fellow Taoists, students, clients, families, and friends who have inspired the writing of this book by their eager desire to understand Pi Gu Chi Kung.

We thank the many contributors essential to this book's final form: the editorial and production staff at Inner Traditions/Destiny Books for their efforts to clarify the text and produce a handsome new edition of the book, and Nancy Yeilding for her line edit of the new edition.

A special thanks goes to our Thai production team: Hirunyathorn Punsan, Sopitnapa Promnon, Udon Jandee, and Suthisa Chaisarn.

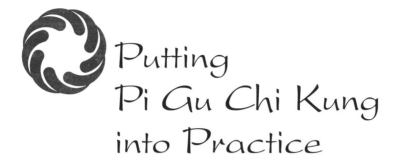

Putting Pi Gu Chi Kung into Practice

The information presented in this book is based on the authors' personal experience and knowledge of Pi Gu and Inner Alchemy. The practices described in this book have been used successfully for thousands of years by Taoists trained by personal instruction. Readers should not undertake the practice without receiving personal transmission and training from a certified instructor of the Universal Healing Tao, since certain of these practices, if done improperly, may cause injury or result in health problems. This book is intended to supplement individual training by the Universal Healing Tao and to serve as a reference guide for these practices. Anyone who undertakes these practices on the basis of this book alone does so entirely at his or her own risk.

The meditations, practices, and techniques described herein are not intended to be used as an alternative or substitute for professional medical treatment and care. If any readers are suffering from illnesses based on physical, mental, or emotional disorders, an appropriate professional health care practitioner or therapist should be consulted. Such problems should be corrected before you start training.

Neither the Universal Healing Tao nor its staff and instructors can be responsible for the consequences of any practice or misuse of the information contained in this book. If the reader undertakes any exercise without strictly following the instructions, notes, and warnings, the responsibility must lie solely with the reader.

This book does not attempt to give any medical diagnosis, treatment, prescription, or remedial recommendation in relation to any human disease, ailment, suffering, or physical condition whatsoever.

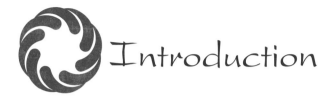 Introduction

Pi Gu is an ancient Taoist, or Chinese, mode of fasting that has been known about and practiced by a small minority of adepts, mainly during spiritual retreats, for some thousands of years. The ancient texts refer to Pi Gu as an "energy fast" or "energizing fast," as the body's energy levels increase while food consumption decreases radically, but without eliminating eating entirely. Experienced Taoists may consume only fruit and water during prolonged meditations lasting months, and the ancients could go without any food or drink at all for long periods (fig. I.1). But

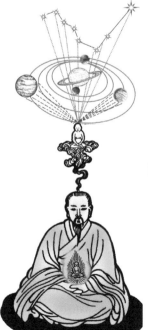

Fig. I.1. Taoist sage

this level of fasting is difficult to fit into our lives today. Mantak Chia has revived the legendary Pi Gu energizing fast and adapted it to our times, making it easy for the modern student of Taoism, or those with weight or health problems, to benefit from it.

Pi Gu (fig. I.2) literally means to "stop eating grains," although some translators would say "stop eating" or "stop eating meat." We can take it to mean in effect to stop eating meat, grains, and processed foods. But Pi Gu does not mean to stop eating altogether; in fact the types of food allowed depend on the level of spiritual practices.

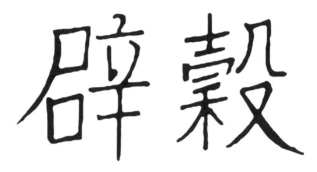

Fig. I.2. Chinese symbol of Pi Gu

We know that if we want to get energy and whatever we need to exist, we have to "spend" something. So we work hard in order to produce or buy food, and then we work to cook the food. But these days you can buy many different sorts of foods or go to many restaurants and other places that serve food. We are spoiled for choice; even gas stations serve hot and cold food and everything is available outside traditional mealtimes (fig. I.3). There is also a lot of "junk" food available, leading to an overconsumption of food, when food should really be a precious asset. So we do not choose raw ingredients and cook them as much as we used to; indeed many people do not know how to shop for raw ingredients or cook at all.

We eat the food, chew it, and digest it, which takes a lot of time. Digestion depends on what sort of food you eat, but it takes from four to six hours. After that your body must absorb the nutrients and the

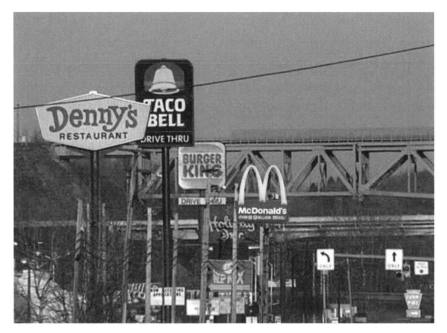

Fig. I.3. Multiple choices for fast food

blood carries them around to distribute them where needed. And we need good air to breathe to keep this system flowing.

When your stomach, liver, spleen, or other members of the digestive system have problems, you do not absorb nutrients well, so you don't obtain optimal energy from your food. You can spend 100 percent of your energy in the form of time and money but if the stomach cannot digest, the nutrients cannot be absorbed. So no matter what you spend, you get poor value for it. It is like spending 100 euros and getting 33 euros worth of use. If the food is only fat and sugar, the body has nothing to feed on. In the short term you are losing out, spending more to get less. This will not lead to better health.

One way to improve the energy from your food consumption is to chew your food better. Pi Gu involves chewing techniques, which ensure that your saliva and food mixture becomes liquid; they also mix in oxygen and nitrogen from the air. This provides the body with material and cosmic energy, perfect building blocks for the body to nourish itself. In this way there is no need to eat as much food, the excess of which turns into waste that is flushed down the toilet.

It is also important to clean out toxins that have built up in your system, like clogged plumbing. This will also help break the cycle of urges for bad food and will get your hormonal and other bodily systems working properly. In this way, you will start to get value for what you spend on food, up to a 100 percent return, or even 120 percent!

There is energy inside of us, which we can call bioelectromagnetic power. The energy outside of us is electromagnetic power. The difference between the two is the *bio* part, which means "life." Each living thing—trees, plants, animals—knows how to use energy. If we can convert the energy from outside then we can use it and will have more energy, or chi.

We can divide the energy from outside in this way: Cosmic Chi from the cosmos, or the creator, the original force; Universal Chi; and Earth Chi. Earth Chi comes from Mother Earth and comes up to us through the soles of our feet, the perineum, and the sexual organs. Universal Chi is all around us in the universe, including all galaxies, and is the chi that feeds all things in nature. The original force is like a spark plug, which provides the spark of fire that, with oxygen, nitrogen, and other nutrients, combusts to give you power, the energy to live on (fig. I.4). Chi is also the end product, the energy that drives the motor. Chi moves; if you move

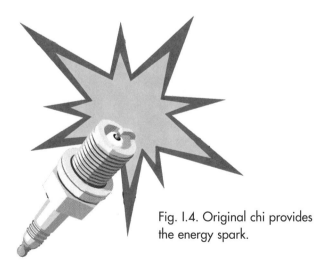

Fig. I.4. Original chi provides the energy spark.

the chi inside of you, the energy will stay longer in you. This is the role of Chi Kung in helping your system get back to working well.

Pi Gu is not a fast in which you stop eating altogether, but one in which your body turns to another energy for nourishment. It is based on eating less as your chi increases. As you advance in the practice, the chi builds up and you eat less and less, but you have so much chi that you are energized. Chi produces chi; that is very important to understand. A person who does not have energy cannot take in other energies. A simple and down-to-earth example can be seen in a dead person, who does not eat any more, so cannot produce chi or take in more chi. When you are able to produce chi for yourself, then you can absorb more chi from elsewhere to help you. By focusing on your "good heart, good mind," and meditating on the circulation of chi in the body, then you can get more chi (fig. I.5). When you get to a higher force, you are

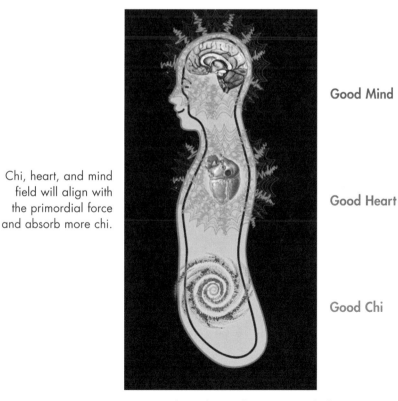

Chi, heart, and mind field will align with the primordial force and absorb more chi.

Good Mind

Good Heart

Good Chi

Fig. I.5. Good Mind, Good Heart, Good Chi

using Cosmic Chi, which has everything you need. As you gradually convert it, then the body naturally cuts down its food intake.

The first chapter of this book describes the development of Pi Gu in the ancient past and its modern validity. Many thousands of Taoist masters have done Pi Gu for long periods without having a body breakdown, but the length of their Pi Gu depended on their chi. However, if you fast for too long, then you can only hope that the body will keep going by itself. Doing Pi Gu in the modern world, we must understand how long is long enough and how to do the fast safely and wisely. That is why we supplement it with some basic foods, as outlined in the second chapter.

Pi Gu is most efficient when used in a spiritual retreat, and indeed the chi generated helps the concentration during the retreat. In chapter 3 we describe in detail how Pi Gu is integrated into the Tao Garden darkroom retreats.

Pi Gu differs from other fasts or fasting diets in three main ways:

1. Pi Gu is *not* a complete fast but does limit food choices for the duration of the fast—mainly eliminating grains, meats, and processed foods, and there is a lot less food eaten overall.
2. The *way* food is eaten is as important as what is eaten: proper chewing is an important part of the Pi Gu diet. This book contains a whole chapter on chewing (chapter 4).
3. Pi Gu is *always* accompanied by Chi Kung meditation practices to draw in more chi from outside the body. Through Chi Kung we have an external source of energy, hence we can eat less without becoming exhausted. We can think of it as spiritual food, and we train ourselves to tap into this other source. These energy meditation practices are highlighted in this book, especially in chapters 5 through 8.

Although Pi Gu is used during spiritual retreats, Master Chia also teaches it during shorter sessions on his world teaching tours, as part of a "Back to Body Wisdom" program. He always incorporates Chi Kung practices, which range from simple to complex, to help digestion, detoxification, and healing. Even moderate following of Pi Gu aids in resetting the body's habits and regaining its natural balance, providing the benefits of weight loss, getting rid of food cravings, and improving both energy levels and digestion, leading to overall health improvements.

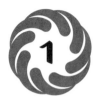

Pi Gu Theory

PI GU DEVELOPMENT

Pi Gu is already a well-experimented and practiced method of fasting, coming from our Taoist ancestors. There is the popularized image of the Taoist hermit sage wandering into the mountains, searching for an appropriate cave, and staying there comfortably for months, drinking only dew from leaves. These Taoists could enter into a state of spontaneous Pi Gu through their Chi Kung and meditational practices and could survive on virtually no food when the body and the digestive system were filled with chi. They initially ate very simple food and then the Pi Gu diet, which could finally be reduced to one Pi Gu pill.

Extracts of the Taoist canon and some old Chinese texts make references to Pi Gu (fig. 1.1). There are a few chi masters today who practice it and who can transmit chi to their students to help them with the fast. The ancient texts always make reference to Inner Alchemy too, and that is why Chi Kung, and the Universal Healing Tao's supreme Inner Alchemy practices in the form of meditations and Chi Kung, are a vital part of Pi Gu.

We can only imagine that some thousands of years ago, a Taoist started fasting, through circumstances or design, and then saw that at a certain level he or she started to be able to turn inward, experiencing a

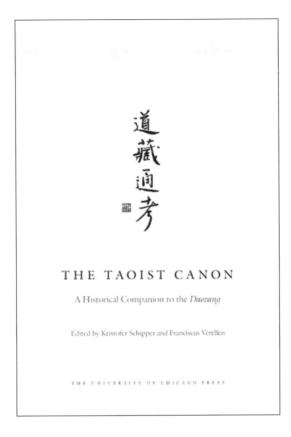

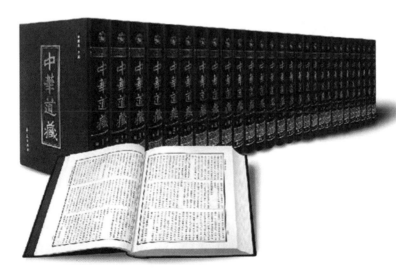

Fig. 1.1. The Taoist canon

level of chi in which the body went into a spontaneous Pi Gu state, as it had tuned in to another source of energy.

Or—since Chinese medicine is mainly based on studying living things—perhaps Pi Gu began with observing turtles, experts in longevity. Taoists love turtles even though they are cold-blooded reptiles. Legend has it that the ancient Taoists studied turtles that were trapped or lived in a seasonal well. When the well would dry up, the turtles were observed coming out every night and staring up at the moon. They could be heard swallowing their saliva, also shown by the position of their outstretched necks (fig. 1.2). They would then bring the neck back in and go back down the well, surviving for many years in this way. This is how saliva elixir was discovered.

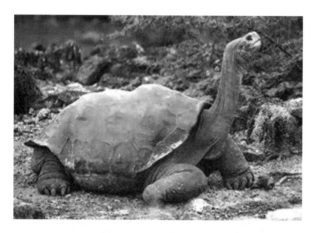

Fig. 1.2. Turtle neck position

Western zoologists have studied bears—we could call them "yogi bears," as they fast when winter comes around. They can stop or freeze bodily functions and hibernate for nearly six months a year. However, they are warm-blooded like us, and when they have babies they have to feed them. It is amazing that they can store fat and convert it to baby food while they are not actually ingesting food.

From these examples we can see that it is possible and important to find a source of energy other than just food. Armed with this knowledge, the Taoists of old could see the point of fasting, and at the same time they saw it as a way to cure the body of certain conditions.

FASTING

Fasting is a traditional spiritual mode; many religions practice forms of fast for spiritual reasons. Christianity has Lent, apparently originating in Jesus's forty days and nights in the desert without food. Muslims practice Ramadan, when they do not eat or drink between sunrise and sunset. Buddha famously experienced fasting when, as Prince Siddhartha, he agreed to fast with an entourage of yogis, until they had achieved enlightenment. The group sat under a tree in that fasting state, with their bodies becoming very thin, to the point of sufferance (fig. 1.3).

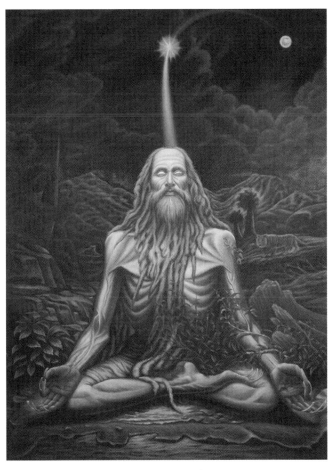

Fig. 1.3. Emaciated yogi

At a certain point Prince Siddhartha observed a man and his grandson going past in a boat. The man was teaching the boy to play an instrument and said, "If you tighten the string too tight, you make a sound but the string might break; if you adjust it just right, it plays great music; but if too slack, you will not have a musical noise." The prince (now the Buddha) heard this as "If it is too tight, your body will break; if too slack, no sound—nothing; but just right, it works; this is the middle path, the middle way." That was his enlightenment (fig. 1.4). He washed, cut his hair, accepted food that a lady offered him, and broke the fast. The yogis were angry he had abandoned their agreement. But he saw no sense in continuing in this absolute fast, having arrived at the middle path conclusion. We can think of Pi Gu as a "middle way" fast.

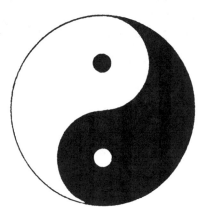

Fig. 1.4. Balance = Middle Way

People meditating in caves need chi, as it is very difficult to find food in caves. One of Master Chia's students told him a story about visiting such a yogi:

I went to the Himalayas, in India, to see the hermits living in caves in the snowy mountains. These yogis meditate to a level where they eat almost nothing, sometimes just sap from trees and water, like the Taoist masters of old.

I saw that one yogi had a pan and gas burner outside his cave. I asked the yogi if I could do anything for him. The yogi said yes, could you go down the mountain to the river with the pan and get some water, as he needed some hot water.

I saw that it was a long way down and back but that there was a lot of snow outside the cave. So to the yogi's astonishment, I filled the pan with snow and boiled it for him. The yogi said he had been there for twenty years and had struggled to go down to the river to get water when he needed it but had never realized that he was surrounded by water up in his cave. He had been so focused on his meditations that this had not come to him. His need of food was virtually nil as he had reached a spiritual level where his body needs had changed. He used chi for nourishment.

However, the yogi's body is not the physical body we are seeking to achieve in Taoist meditations. Taoists believe in keeping the physical body strong in order to provide more chi to feed our souls and spirits to advance in our spiritual practices, which we believe we are here on this earth to do. Fasting with spiritual aims turns our focus away from the body, which has stopped many of its usual functions, toward the mind. Turning the focus inward in this way allows more reflection and awareness of other things.

On a lower plane, there are also fasting methods for losing weight or for turning the body away from an excessive lifestyle. There are also adapted methods, such as what is known as "the 5/2," which involves fasting for two days of the week and eating normally for the other five. This intermittent fasting can provide an achievable alternative for someone who must pursue a busy life at the same time. In any case, digestion itself consumes much energy and some of this energy is available when the body is not consuming food.

DANGERS OF FASTING TOO LONG

The Taoists discovered that you cannot reverse things immediately. We have seen many people on fasts whose bodies get into real physical trouble and sometimes never recover. A common problem, from which many spiritual adepts (including Master Chia's own Taoist master) have suffered, is gallbladder failure, usually due to gallstones.

Why do we have a gallbladder? The gallbladder's main function is to store bile produced by the liver. The liver is a multifunctional organ that produces over five hundred bodily chemicals in a day, including bile, digestive juices, and cholesterol. When food goes down to the stomach, the liver starts producing the chemicals necessary for digestion. When its other functions are in high demand, the liver's bile production is set aside. Then, when no food is arriving, most likely at night, bile production is resumed. When the liver produces bile it sends it to the gallbladder to be stored.

When a person is fasting to the point of abstaining from food, the liver can go into overdrive on its bile production, as its other digestive products are not needed. The gallbladder no longer needs to send bile out to be used in digestion and must store what quickly becomes an excess. Gallstones, which are impacted bile, can form, harden, and consequently enlarge and become inflamed. The gallbladder duct can get blocked and infection can set in. In serious cases the gallbladder has to be removed.

Hormone Balance and Fasting Effects in the Body

The body's complex system of hormones can also become very disrupted during fasting. The thyroid gland controls body metabolism and fasting can cause the thyroid to slow down; this will inevitably slow down digestion as the body will try to conserve body mass. However, it will also lead to a reduction in muscle mass as amino acids are used as a source of energy instead of nutrients.

Production of the stress hormone cortisol will increase as the body reacts to fasting by going into a panic or starvation mode. This can lead to mental and physical trauma. These effects typically lead to feeling physically weak. The immune system of the body will also be weakened. This is the importance of Pi Gu as a middle path. It does not represent the same physical risks to the body of stopping alimentation altogether, which can create imbalances.

MECHANICS OF EATING— CHEWING AND THE STOMACH

The stomach does not have teeth and cannot do the "predigestive work" of the mouth and saliva. The teeth are in the mouth and that is where chewing needs to take place, with the other parts of the mouth helping with mixing and movement, like in a mixer (fig. 1.5). The body starts digestive juice production (fig. 1.6) as soon as you start chewing

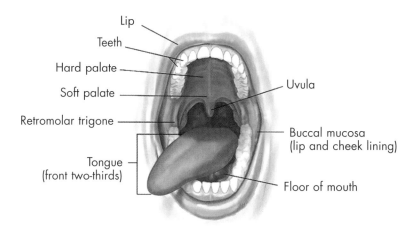

Fig. 1.5. Anatomy of the mouth

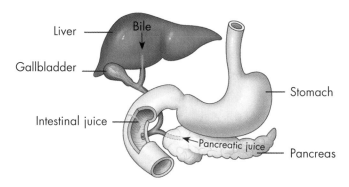

Fig. 1.6. Stomach and digestive juices

the food, but of course you need a certain amount of chewing to get enough juices to work on the mouthful of food. Otherwise the work of the stomach does not take place correctly.

The stomach (fig. 1.7) is a muscular bag whose job is to mix food with the digestive juices produced by the body, which enable it to be broken down into nutrients and waste.

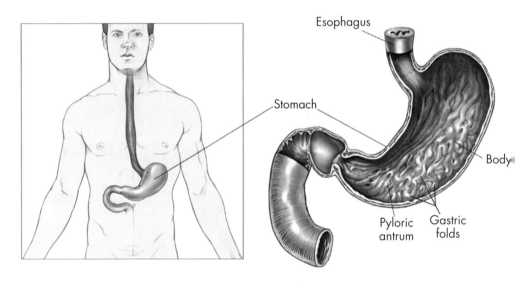

Fig. 1.7. Stomach

The stomach can expand to five times its own size. So if one eats a huge meal, the stomach will happily expand. But when you mix ingredients together, you need some space in the receptacle in order to mix them thoroughly. Take a washing machine or a mixer like a kitchen mixer or a cement mixer: if they are filled to the brim, mixing cannot occur. Overeating will expand the stomach until it eventually retains a larger volume, and continuing to overeat will impede good mixing. The stretching of the stomach will weaken its elasticity, and it will operate with less efficiency (fig. 1.8).

Swallowing food that is not chewed up sufficiently to go into the stomach and then filling the stomach up too much—that is, eating too much—results in indigestion and then gas. Stomach gas can be uncom-

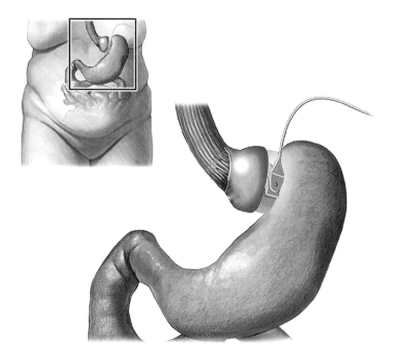

Fig. 1.8. The bloated stomach in this illustration has been fitted
with a gastric band in a surgical attempt to slow consumption of
food and reduce overall food intake.

fortable and stretch the stomach even more. The food mixture gets sent
further on its way in a state that does not suit the intestines. The intestines need the food digested into a nano state so that the nutrients can
be absorbed into the blood stream. When the food particles are too big
the intestines cannot make proper use of the nourishment.

While the stomach can expand when required to up to five times its
original size, after a while it will not go back to its original size. Tackling obesity by surgical stomach reduction is becoming commonplace
now, particularly in the U.S. However, this bariatric surgery has been
producing some strange side effects. It changes the way that the body
processes alcohol, making the person inebriate within minutes of swallowing alcohol. It also may change the person's body chemistry, facili-
tating dependency on alcohol. There is currently a study at St. Olav's

University in Norway to further investigate this worrying progression of new alcoholics among postsurgery patients. A society that has reached such an extreme surely has to rethink its relationship with eating, and its ways of tackling the problem.

OVEREATING AND OBESITY

Overeating is a problem in Western society and many thriving countries around the world, in contrast to countries where there is strife, famine, and starvation. In the countries where we overeat, food is cheap, but the cheapest food is often the wrong food for our bodies. Processed foods and junk food restaurants add many chemicals to the food so that it smells good, tastes good, and prompts us to keep eating it. But the stomach does not always like it; we are pleasing the tongue but making life difficult for the stomach. "Wrong" foods are consumed because of cravings and poor food choices. Nutrients cannot be absorbed properly; waste does not flow out easily; toxins build up.

During his work in the United States, Master Chia was amazed by a visit to a "Buffet City" in Chicago. In an $18 "all you can eat" buffet restaurant, he witnessed the enormous quantities of food that people were eating. This included children who were drinking king-size glasses of sodas with their large portions of fattening food, and then going back for refills. The majority of the diners were very overweight (fig. 1.9 and fig. 1.10). This scene was a shock for Master Chia's party of Chi Kung practitioners, but it is not an uncommon scene. Obesity is becoming a major problem.

Key Facts on Obesity and Overweight from the World Health Organization—March 2013

Worldwide obesity has nearly doubled since 1980.

In 2008, more than 1.4 billion adults, 20 and older, were overweight. Of these, over 200 million men and nearly 300 million women were obese.

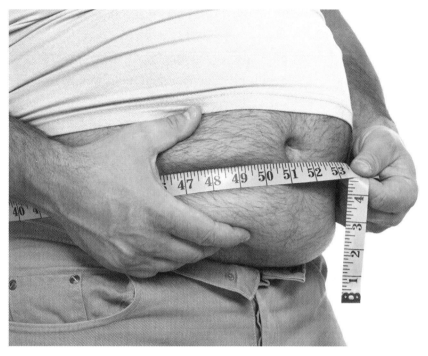

Fig. 1.9. Overweight adult

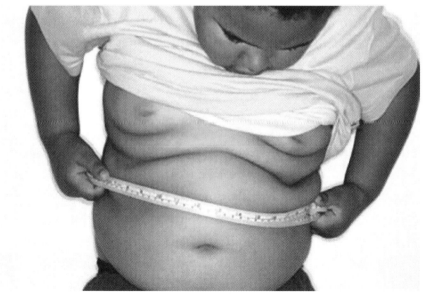

Fig. 1.10. Obesity affects more and more children.

5% of adults aged 20 and over were overweight in 2008, and 11% were obese.

65% of the world's population live in countries where overweight and obesity kills more people than underweight.

More than 40 million children under the age of five were overweight in 2011.

Obesity is preventable.

The body has always known that fat is necessary for survival and it will easily absorb it into the small intestines. Fat is absorbed whether you chew it well or not, particularly animal fat. Fat will be stored everywhere in the body; if it is stored in significant excess it will eventually block blood vessels, the liver, and the heart. This is a major killer. And recent research suggests that food additives and antibiotics in meat are aiding and abetting unusual weight gain.

When the body is congested with fat, the stem cells like to gather in the abdomen, their natural place, but they cannot travel to repair or replace damaged cells due to the blocked routes. They want to help so they begin to store fat. Doctors discovered that they could extract abdominal fat and centrifuge out the fat, then the cells could turn back to stem cells and fix many problems. But this is not a solution available to many.

WEIGHT LOSS AND PI GU

Taoist wisdom can help weight problems that have become endemic to our society. Weight loss is a side effect of Pi Gu, making it of huge potential interest. We have been able to study the effects of the inclusion of Pi Gu in Universal Tao darkroom retreats and other workshops for some years.

Students have lost an average of ten pounds a week practicing Pi Gu during the darkroom retreats. Whether they are on retreat for one, two, or three weeks, students do not generally report feeling hungry during the experience or feeling weak from the weight loss. Students who continued Pi Gu on their own reported continual weight loss. Those students welcomed this side effect of Pi Gu as they were happy to lose some weight and reset their bodies' eating habits.

THE BENEFIT OF EVEN CUTTING DOWN BY 10 PERCENT

Mantak Chia states in his Pi Gu class lecture, "When we have enough chi, the body will need less food. It will be good for us and for the world if we cut food needed by even only 10 percent." Of course, if the overweight cut down their food intake by 10 percent, there would be financial consequences in the food industry. There would be job losses in factories, as production would have to drop by 10 percent, and effects in food retailing, distribution, supermarkets, and restaurants.

In fact it might initially seem bad for the economy. However, it would be accompanied by tremendous health benefits for society, and the health care budgets for dealing with overeating would go down. Recent health studies show that for the obese and overweight, shedding only 5 percent of body weight can significantly reduce the risks of diabetes and heart disease.

PI GU FOSTERS ENLIGHTENMENT

During Pi Gu fasting there is also a raising of consciousness and higher awareness. Energy levels increase not only from the energy saved from the digestion system but also from the extra chi absorbed by the body in the Chi Kung practices such as "eating the cosmos"—chewing air and liquefying the oxygen and nitrogen. As the Chi Kung practices reach a high level, the stomach is filled with chi, and more energy than usual is felt.

Some Chi Kung practices activate sexual hormones from the

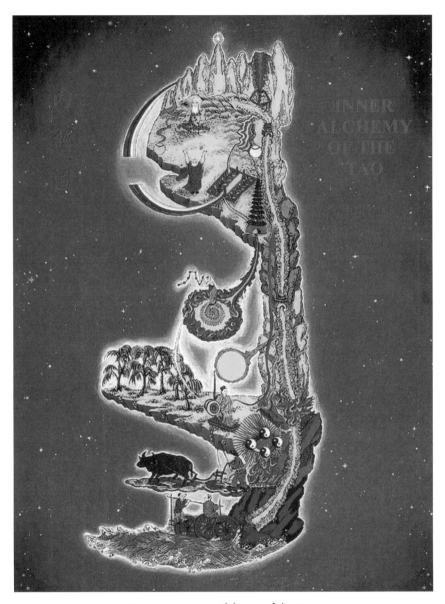

Fig. 1.11. Inner Alchemy of the Tao

The Pi Gu experience as described in this book supports
realization of the Five Enlightenments of the Tao.

testicles, nipples, and genitals, which go to the brain, stimulating the secretions to flow down like nectar, or elixir, also known as the fountain of youth. The increase in chi also fosters gaining enlightenment through Inner Alchemy meditations (see fig. 1.11 on page 22), for example, the Kan and Li meditations practiced in the darkroom retreat.

The Five Enlightenments of the Tao

In the First Enlightenment we realize that we have a basic soul and spirit.

In the Second Enlightenment we go deeper and realize we have a baby soul and baby spirit or a child soul and a child spirit. We realize that we have children and we must take care of them.

The Third Enlightenment is when we say, "I want to be responsible and raise my soul and spirit."

The Fourth Enlightenment is when we go deeper still, understanding more with wisdom and knowledge. We realize that no one can have power over our soul and spirit, not any faith, religion, or God. "I have a free spirit and I must choose my own way." The Tao says that if we realize we have a free spirit, no one can control our soul and spirit. We are free.

Now when we have a baby or child soul and spirit what are we going to do? If we have made up our mind that we will raise our soul and spirit and we are determined to do it, we have the Fifth Enlightenment. Combining all of the above, we begin to have the Greatest Enlightenment.

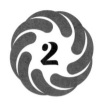

Changing Your Diet through the Pi Gu Experience

Mantak Chia has made an important commitment to researching and promoting Pi Gu training. After much research and personal practice, he first introduced Pi Gu into the Tao Garden 2010 darkroom retreat program (presented in the next chapter). He had found that if people followed this Pi Gu program for twenty-one days, then their diet changed naturally afterward. There are already changes after one week, but the longer people do it, the more long-term the changes are and the higher the energy raised.

As we have said, Pi Gu is not a complete fast. The next chapter goes into great detail about Pi Gu in the Universal Healing Tao darkroom retreats. Here we present only a general outline of the foods and beverages that are included as part of the Pi Gu fasting regimen.

Pi Gu Beverages

- Chlorophyll drink
- Ginger tea
- Mulberry tea

- Native Legend Tea* (for lymphatic detox)
- Nature's T Infusion* (a natural detox of the lungs and digestive system)
- Immortal Tea (also known as Jiaogulan or *Gynostemma pentaphyllum*)

Pi Gu Foods
Fruits

- Apple
- Pear
- Watermelon
- Tomato
- Juju berries
- Goji berries

Nuts, Seeds, Beans

- Steamed peanuts
- Walnuts
- Steamed edamame beans
- Sesame seeds

Other

- Steamed egg white

In addition, we also serve our own especially formulated Pi Gu pill, an elixir ball of herbs and fruit, including Chinese plums or prunes, goji berries, or other berries, walnuts, peanuts, black sesame seeds, herbs, pepper, hot spices, and dates, ground together and mixed with a little honey. These are available at Tao Garden at certain times of the year—during darkroom retreats—and can be ordered from Tao Garden.

By following the Pi Gu fast, the body will refine its choices naturally and will start to choose simpler food. Sometimes the food you used to

---

*These teas are special formulations prepared by a supplier for Universal Healing Tao. They are available in the Pakua Clinic at Tao Garden Health Spa and Resort.

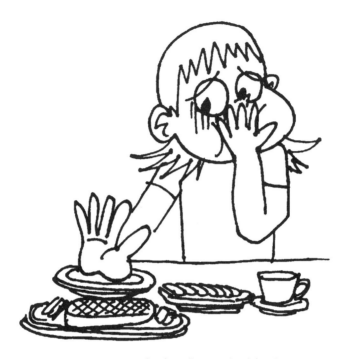

Fig. 2.1. Your body will reject bad food.

like will even make you feel sick when you try to eat it again (fig. 2.1). There are people who vomit as the body reacts strongly to what it does not want in its system.

PANIC IN THE BODY

When dieting, the body can go into panic mode. This parallels what takes place in society if there is a situation in which food supplies are disrupted, such as during strikes or shortages or more serious problems. There is a panic and people "panic-buy" food and stockpile it (fig. 2.2). When the problem is over, they have often forgotten what they have stored and where.

The body can do something similar after an extreme diet or fast: it can feel disrupted and panic. The body starts broadcasting the wrong information within itself, leading you to start eating fat and sugar because those are the basic staples that it needs. It will start

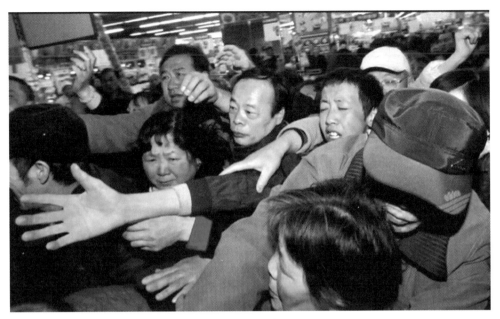

Fig. 2.2. Panic buying

storing those things. Then, after digestion, the body will tell you it needs more sugars and fats. This is misinformation or misinterpretation, as the body will not know what it really needs. That is why the majority of people who fast and diet end up being heavier some time afterward.

This is one reason that the body needs to be detoxed before you change your eating habits. The Pi Gu regime works much more efficiently if it is accompanied by detox. This is especially evident with people who have a smoking or drug problem. Their chances of getting away from their cravings are much higher if they combine detox with their Pi Gu. A system in this state needs fourteen days of detoxification before it can reset itself. You need to cleanse the body and chew very well to set it on its right path again.

Also, if you chew well, you will start eating smaller quantities. When the mass of food you are eating gets bigger with the extra saliva added to it, the pineal gland will give the message that you have had enough much sooner.

TOXINS AND CRAVINGS

The pineal gland can create cravings to eat or not to eat certain things. A craving generally means that your body needs certain sorts of nutrients that you are not ingesting. However, our theory is that when there are too many toxins in the body, it becomes confused about what it really needs, like an overtired child who will say "no" to everything her helpful parents are suggesting. The toxins are preventing the senses from working properly to signal actual needs. There is usually emotional confusion too. Addictions to sugars and other ingredients in foods can result in cravings too.

We need something, but the brain no longer knows what, and the body is too toxic and too emotional and so makes demands (fig. 2.3).

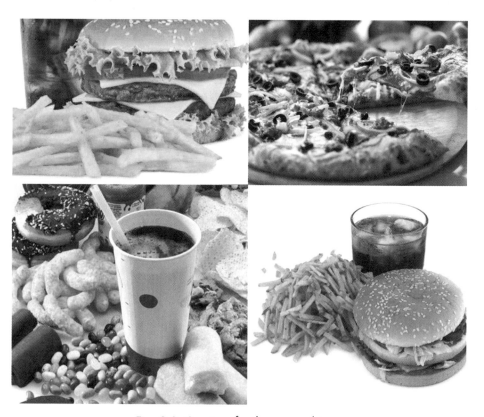

Fig. 2.3. Cravings for the wrong things

The pituitary gland says "what do you want?" but the brain doesn't know. Confusion reigns, but the basic body needs are fat and sugar, so that is what it will ask for!

If you follow your cravings, you will continue to eat the wrong foods and make the problem worse. As you are not getting the nutrients that the body needs, you will continue to eat in search of them. That is, of course, a recipe for gaining more weight. People who are already overweight and lacking in energy seem to crave junk food and sugars, which is exactly a downward spiral and will make their problem worse.

Removing Emotional Toxins with the Six Healing Sounds

Cravings are often associated with emotional problems. We confuse our bodies by having so many emotions going around inside (fig. 2.4).

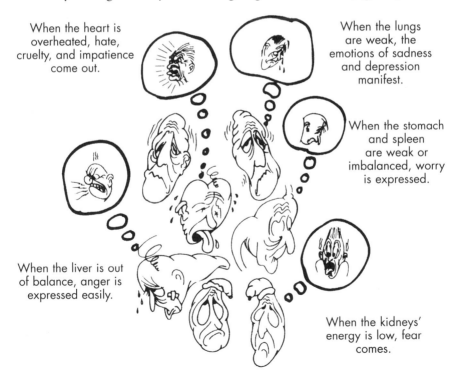

When the heart is overheated, hate, cruelty, and impatience come out.

When the lungs are weak, the emotions of sadness and depression manifest.

When the stomach and spleen are weak or imbalanced, worry is expressed.

When the liver is out of balance, anger is expressed easily.

When the kidneys' energy is low, fear comes.

Fig. 2.4. Emotions upset organs.

Taoists use the Six Healing Sounds exercise to eliminate emotional toxins. Detoxing our negative emotions with the Six Healing Sounds cuts the link between, for example, feeling unloved and eating chocolate (fig. 2.5). (The Six Healing Sounds practice is detailed in

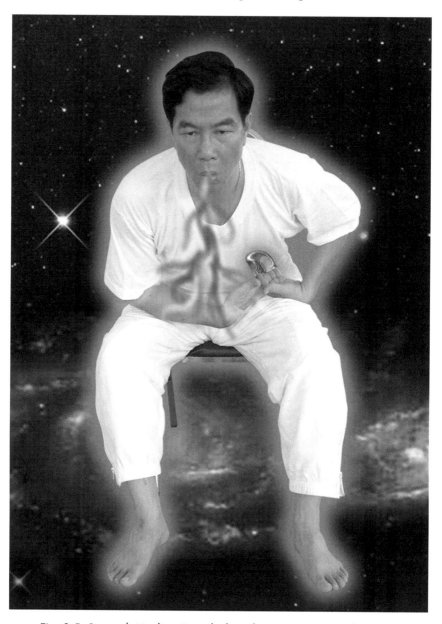

Fig. 2.5. Stomach Healing Sound—breathing out worry and anxiety

our book *The Six Healing Sounds: Taoist Techniques for Balancing Chi* and also in *Basic Practices of the Universal Healing Tao*, pages 40–45; see "Recommended Reading" at the back of this book). Taoists also use the Inner Smile, which replaces negative emotions by smiling in positive, loving ones.

RELIEVING CRAVINGS BY MASSAGE

Massaging certain points of the body will also help to release cravings.

 ### Massage the Windy City and Jade Pillow

The points to use are at the back of the head, shown in the diagram below. The middle of this area is called the Jade Pillow; on either side of it is the Windy City (fig. 2.6).

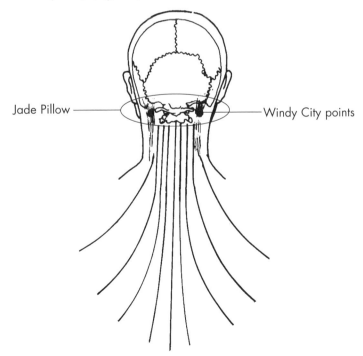

Fig. 2.6. Rub the Windy City points on the back of head.

1. Rub the Windy City points with your hands, turning with your thumbs or fingers until you find an area that hurts. This means you have hit the spot!

2. Continue rubbing until you feel something clearing up and energy going into your brain. When you have cleaned out this area, it will no longer feel so sensitive; the pain should stop.

3. Now place your fingers in the middle of the Jade Pillow, which is connected to the small brain and the main brain. Continue to clear out this area in the same way by rubbing it until there is no longer pain. The energy will be flowing, so just rest, feeling that your brain is clearer.

 ## Massage the Collar Bone Points

The two craving points behind the collar bone will be painful too, due to a build up of toxins (fig. 2.7). The head is heavier than the neck, so the neck and shoulders can feel a lot of strain from supporting the head. As we are often leaning forward, or slightly to one side, this makes

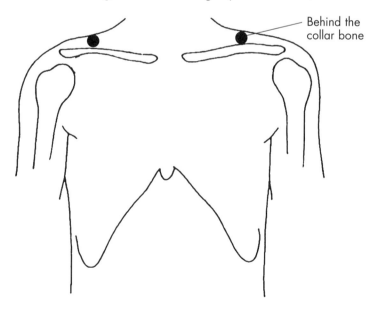

Fig. 2.7. Massage points behind the collar bone

remaining perfectly balanced difficult for the neck and shoulders. The cravings points send signals into the brain: if they are the wrong signals, it confuses the brain.

Take one point at a time or both together, with a finger of the opposite hand, and press down on it.

 ## Massage Points along the Gall Bladder Line

The Gall Bladder line continues down the body to the feet. Cravings can come from here, so search for the points and you will know when you have found them because they will be painful. The smart phone, or the un-smart phone, pushes the shoulders out of line and also sends wrong signals to the brain. Holding it to one ear for a long phone call is unbalancing and tends to make the body lean to one side (fig. 2.8). Holding it between the shoulder and the ear strains our straight shoulder line. This is a common problem, and this misalignment is

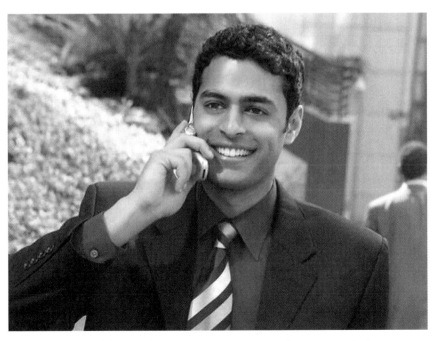

Fig. 2.8. Holding a phone to your ear extensively creates imbalance.

another reason for food cravings, so bear it in mind and correct the body position.

1. Massage down the Gall Bladder line, looking for painful places. In fact you will probably find pain on many points along it (fig. 2.9). One side is usually more painful, in which case try to train yourself to sit straighter.

2. When sitting for a while, make a point of stopping to open the chest more. We often forget to do things like that when working or absorbed.

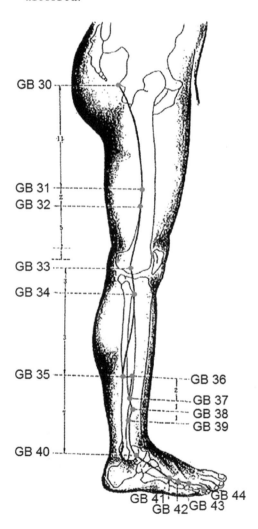

Fig. 2.9. Gall Bladder line

TREATING EATING DISORDERS WITH PI GU

We have to be able to generate our own chi before we can get more chi. The Universal Healing Tao practices can help rebalance the organs' chi while transforming negative emotions. At Tao Garden, people suffering from eating disorders are initially helped to exercise more, even people suffering from anorexia. In the case of anorexia sufferers, we have to get them to feel and appreciate body normality before investigating why they cannot eat.

 ## Shaking

This simple exercise is good for someone who is anorexic or has burnout or other fatigue syndromes. In fact, it is good for everyone, as it alone will strengthen the digestive system and get rid of toxins by circulating blood and energy. A tired person can do it as slowly and gently as he likes.

1. Stand up with knees flexed, lumbar rounded, and sacrum tucked in.
2. Then move up and down, gently shaking the body all over (see fig. 2.10 on page 36).

 ## Smile to the Lower Tan Tien

When working on food and stomach issues, a good beginning is to start by relaxing the senses down to the lower tan tien and smiling into it (see fig. 2.11 on page 37).

NUTRITIONAL APPROACH TO BURN-OUT SYNDROME AND CANCER

Burn-out syndrome is an umbrella name given to many health problems that leave people tired all or most of the time. Give exhausted people enough real nutrition and they can start to fight back, but what if their bodies can no longer take in nutrients properly?

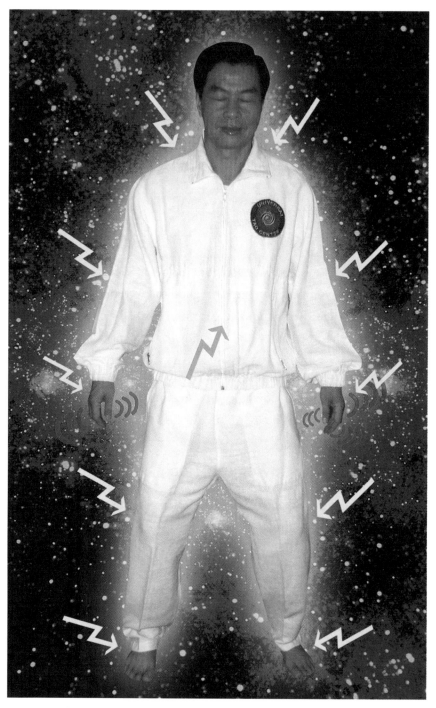

Fig. 2.10. Shaking all over

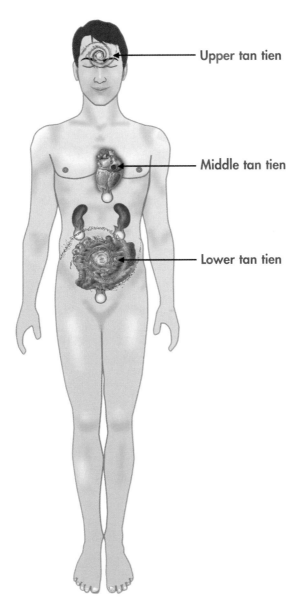

Upper tan tien

Middle tan tien

Lower tan tien

Fig. 2.11. Relaxing the senses down to the lower tan tien

Stress creates a lot of mucous in the body, which then blocks the digestive system. Necessary nutrients are no longer absorbed easily, but fat and sugar remain easily absorbed. Low energy is a consequence. In

Tao Garden we treat this condition by initially detoxing: first colon cleansing and perhaps Chi Nei Tsang and other techniques. Then we feed the patients with the right nutrition and the state of fatigue starts to lift.

We use the same basic approach to cancer patients. Cancer makes the whole body stressed such that it cannot absorb nutrients properly. We have 50 trillion cells, and probably only 1 billion or 50 million cancer cells. The cancer cells are still our cells, so our soldier cells do not kill them, thinking that they are our brothers and sisters.

The cancer cells act like spoiled children; when you eat something they like, they grab it first. It is as if they want to build something in the middle of the road, and they do just that in our body. The other cells get tired and the whole body suffers; this results in much stress and poor absorption of food. The cancer cells thrive on this, so we work to find a set of foods that they do not like but that the other cells need, to starve the cancer cells and build up the body again.

Energy Drink

In Tao Garden we offer a morning energy booster drink that is a meal in itself. It is used as treatment for patients with fatigue syndromes or burnout. It includes:

- Green coffee or green tea
- Protein and hormones extracted from soya
- Calcium and magnesium, chelated together so that the body can use them
- Noni juice

Master Chia travels with this energy drink himself during his world tours, as he cannot be sure where, when, and what he will be eating.

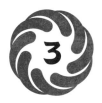

Pi Gu in the Darkroom Retreats at Tao Garden

Master Chia introduced Pi Gu into his darkroom retreat to facilitate the meditations, while at the same time promoting self-healing of the body and resetting of the body system. The construction of the darkroom and the offering of darkroom retreats at Tao Garden make the significant benefits of darkness available to students of the Universal Healing Tao.

Complete darkness enables the body and mind to undergo a series of intense transformations, profoundly changing the sensory sensibilities of the brain. The body is deprived of all visual reference. Sounds begin to fall away as we lose contact with the external world and turn the senses inward. The effect of darkness is to shut down major cortical centers in the brain, depressing mental and cognitive functions in the higher brain centers. Emotional and feeling states are enhanced, especially the sense of smell and the finer senses of psychic perception.

While the darkness meditations influence each person uniquely, depending on their maturity and stage of spiritual development, most people, even beginners, receive great benefits, which may include the following:

- Relaxation: catching up on sleep and allowing the eyes to recuperate from the overstimulation of our visual world, as well as releasing the grip of mental concerns, plans, and agendas and simply letting the energies settle.
- Emotional release: memories and deep-stored emotions linked with past events, as well as stress from particular projects, can present themselves and be swept away by the darkness.
- Advanced practitioners may experience lucid dreaming and a state of continuous consciousness, in which there is no break in conscious awareness; dreams often take the form of teachings or participation in great mythological stories.
- The Taoist secrets of love and Healing Love become very active, making work with sexual energies and creativity easier and more powerful.
- Meditation can continue through sleeping and nonsleeping hours.
- Eventually, the awareness of the Source, the spirit, the soul awakens within. The light appears.

THE TAO GARDEN DARKROOM
RETREAT CENTER

The darkroom retreat building at Tao Garden is a very modern yet comfortable equivalent of the Taoist hermit cave in the mountains (fig. 3.1).

Master Chia decided to adapt a condominium block after visiting many caves in his search for a suitable place to hold a darkroom retreat. It was very difficult to find a cave that did not have damp, mold, insects, snakes, centipedes, or scorpions. The condominium block allows enough space—with bathrooms, bedrooms, and a large central meditation hall—for a large group of students to be comfortable while meditating or practicing Chi Kung for one to three weeks in total darkness.

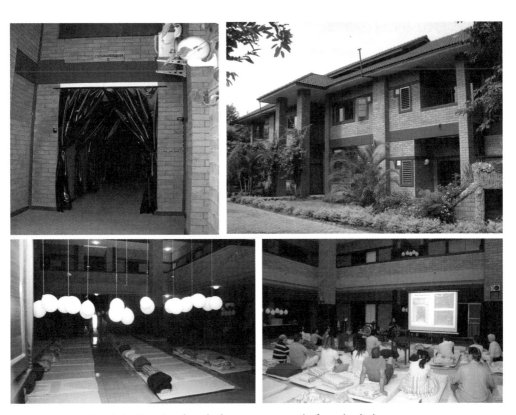

Fig. 3.1. Tao Garden darkroom retreat—before the lights go out

There is space for each participant to have a mattress in the central hall, plus a private or shared bedroom with ensuite bathroom in the rooms around the hall. The layout makes navigating in the dark comparatively easy. A typical first evening will be spent with dimmed lights on while participants familiarize themselves with the building and their own private and class space. They are then able to safely negotiate these spaces in the dark throughout the retreat.

The building is adapted by being covered in material that blacks out all light. A powerful and hygienic air circulation system makes up for the closed and covered windows. Tao Garden staff wear night vision glasses, which enable them to serve participants their Pi Gu meals and drinks in the teaching hall and tend to duties to keep the retreat going in comfort.

Master Chia attends many of the meals, especially breakfast. As well as encouraging chewing, and therefore making it easier for the students to pace themselves, he also gives explanations of Pi Gu and the meditations and answers questions. And he helps induce the Pi Gu state by personally transmitting chi to the students.

PREPARATIONS FOR
THE DARKROOM RETREAT

When students apply to attend the darkroom sessions at Tao Garden, there are prerequisites of a certain level of spiritual practices as necessary background to be able to follow the meditations. If they have been studying the Universal Healing Tao system, then their progression through the practices will show if they are ready for the darkroom experience. If their experience is not from the UHT system, it is essential for the darkroom retreat organizers to understand each student's background in meditation.

Detoxification

One essential and often neglected point when considering fasting is first cleansing the body of built-up toxins and retained waste products. Not many fasts recommend detoxing first. However, the body always has toxins in it and the body systems are built to constantly shift the toxins out. If these systems slow down and stop, due to the absence of food input, there is a big risk that the toxins will build up. The body is no longer able to shift the waste products out in the normal way. This can result in health issues. That is why we recommend some form of detoxification prior to the darkroom retreat.

Before starting the darkroom retreat you can tell the body to reduce food and stick only to the essentials. Give up grains, processed foods, alcohol, caffeine, rich food, and any excesses.

It is also desirable to arrive at Tao Garden early enough to do some organ and colon cleansing before the retreat starts, unless you have been

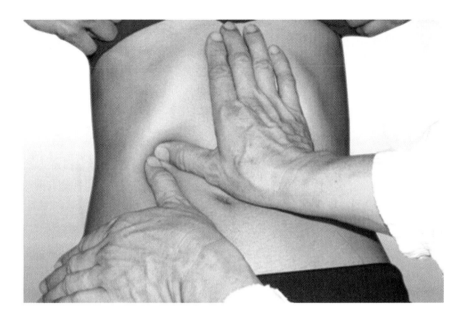

Fig. 3.2. Chi Nei Tsang detoxifies the digestive organs.

able to do this at home. A day or two are needed to acclimatize from a long-haul flight, so doing colon cleansing and the Chi Nei Tsang organ massage at Tao Garden is very practical. Colon cleansing can be in the form of taking laxatives and fiber or colonic hydrotherapy. Chi Nei Tsang massage is a Taoist massage that works directly on the abdomen, vital organs, and emotions (fig. 3.2). The deep massage releases tension and promotes energy and blood flow, which helps the body to expel accumulated toxins. Chi Nei Tsang also includes techniques that work on all of the body's systems and it therefore improves overall health (see fig. 3.3 on page 44).

Chi Nei Tsang treatments can also be given in the darkroom retreat during the afternoon breaks if your body needs some healing (see fig. 3.4 on page 44). If you start with some detoxification beforehand, the cleansing process will continue during the darkroom retreat.

Once in the darkroom, the detoxification continues. Previously, students in the darkroom were given the choice of eating either Pi Gu style

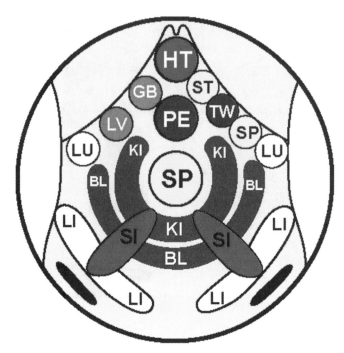

Fig. 3.3. Chi Nei Tsang organ massage locations

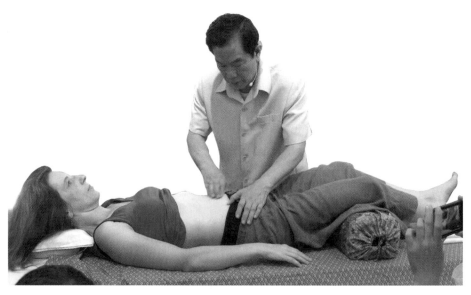

Fig. 3.4. Master Chia teaching Chi Nei Tsang

or light but normal meals. However, everyone elected to follow the Pi Gu option, so this has now become part of the experience for all. Some students have informed us of medical or eating problems, and we have adapted the regime for them.

In Tao Garden we have adopted a system of teas served during and between meals. For many years we did research on detox herbs and products and invested a lot of resources into developing our own system. However, we have found a supplier who has done even more research than we have, and we have been very impressed by their results. So now we use their range of detox teas. We use them in the darkroom and in our Tao Garden spa diets, and many people throughout the world order them directly from us, as we have adapted them into a complete cleansing system.*

PARASITES

A recent documentary on the Discovery Channel showed that parasites give us "orders." Even though they are simple cells, they can occupy our brain and nerves and tell us what to do. They are self-propagating, multiplying in their host's body to pass on generations of themselves.

Master Chia's Taoist master always said that you had to get rid of parasites before they killed you. To put it simply: they are smaller than our red blood cells, and it is difficult to get rid of them even with medicine (see fig. 3.5 on page 46). And the medicines that can be effective in killing them are quite strong, with possible side effects. Even in that case, the parasites can lay eggs before they die, and the eggs are not killed off.

The white blood cells cannot act against the eggs until they hatch out. At that point our army of white blood cells moves to the area, which creates lumps or blockages in our body. The blockages stop the blood from flowing well and prevent the cells from receiving nourishment. Plaque is created, which blocks the capillaries; the parasites hide

---

*For information on ordering detox teas please e-mail the Tao Gardens Health Spa and Retreat at either info@tao-garden.com or taogarden@hotmail.com.

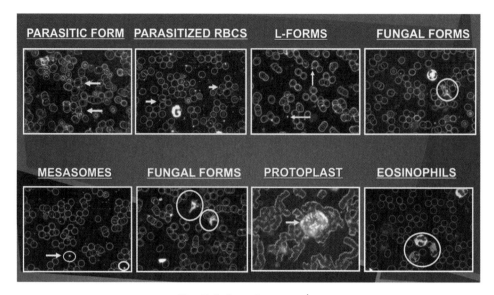

Fig. 3.5. Parasite examples

behind the plaque and attack the white blood cells while building their empire (fig. 3.6). If the blood does not flow correctly, the army and police protection units of our bodies cannot go in and act. So the problems build up.

The cells start to die. The parasite embryos, which are very small, smaller than the cells, get in behind the blockages; their shells stay in place to protect them until they are ready to hatch. The surrounding cells start to nourish them and our white blood cells are more or less helpless to stop them. They grow and multiply, taking weak or dying cells as food. They take over as the area becomes weaker and weaker. This is the beginning of disease. The cells no longer listen to body commands, as they have become disconnected from the natural order. That is the work of parasites in the body.

This is why we have made parasite detoxification a part of the cleansing process in the darkroom. Instead of using strong medicine to kill parasites, we use herbs whose taste and smell they do not like, including powdered walnut hulls, pumpkin seeds, fenugreek seeds, garlic, black pepper, common knotgrass, hyssop, peppermint, thyme, and fennel. When your body is impregnated with this smell and taste, the

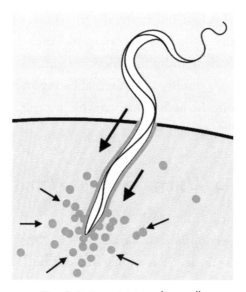

Fig. 3.6. Parasite invading cell

parasites will leave. Upon leaving the body, they will die immediately. A parasite detox tea made up of these herbs is generally served in the morning in the darkroom, before breakfast. A gel capsule containing these herbs, Paraway, is also available at Tao Gardens.

FLUSHING THE THREE WORMS

Ancient Taoists believed that we are born with "Three Worms," or three "Death Bringers," in our bodies, one in each of the three tan tiens, or "fields of energy," located in the third eye area, the heart center area, and the navel area, respectively. As the metaphorical opposites of the Three Pure Ones (positive energies from the Pole Star that dissolve energetic blockages), the Three Worms create emotional, mental, and physical mischief: Peng Ju attacks the upper tan tien; it blocks chi flow to the head and causes overattachment to things that reward the material senses, such as delicious foods or beautiful music and artwork. Peng Zhi attacks the middle tan tien; it blocks chi flow to the heart and causes overattachment to wealth and status and to heightened emotions, such as joy and anger. Peng Jiaou attacks the lower tan tien; it blocks chi flow to the Sexual Palace and causes overattachment to lust and addictions (figs. 3.7 and 3.8). It is necessary to expel these metaphorical worms from the body in order to achieve enlightenment, longevity, and immortality. Ancient Taoists believed that eating grains encourages the worms to remain in the body, which is why "no grains" is a central element of Pi Gu.

Meditation Using the Three Worms

1. Begin this meditation with the Inner Smile (as detailed in our books *The Inner Smile* and *Basic Practices of the Universal Healing Tao,* pages 16–18; see "Recommended Reading" at the back of the book).

2. Become aware of the knots and blockages that are closing down the three tan tiens. These knots and blockages correspond to defilements by the Three Worms.

3. Now, using your imagination, create a multisensory impression of the Three Worms, giving shape to these defilements before breathing out all toxins from the body.

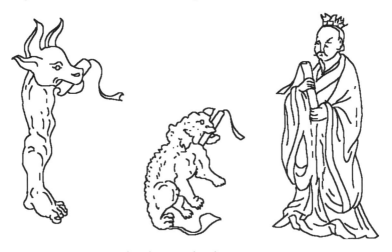

Fig. 3.7. The Three Malevolent Worms: Peng Ju, Peng Zhi, and Peng Jiaou

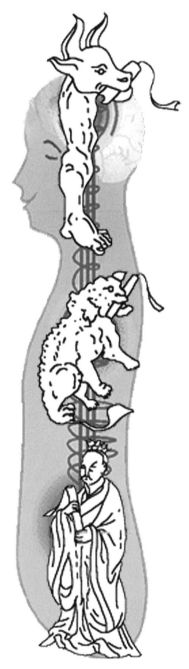

Fig. 3.8. Peng Ju, Peng Zhi, and Peng Jiaou,
corresponding to defilement of the three tan tiens

Certain herbs and Golden Elixir help to flush out the Three Worms (see chapter 8, "Golden Elixir Chi Kung").

Many ancient Taoist theories have eventually found Western scientific support. Could it be that the Three Worms is one of them? There has been much research recently into gut microbes and suggestions that the trillions of billions of microbes we all have in our intestines can control our behavior, our lives, and our bodies. In a similar vein, there have been recent scientific findings on parasites that can control the mind.

Our gut biome can alter the way we store fat, our response to hormones and glucose in the blood, and our desire to eat certain things. "Fecal transfer" is becoming a medicalized intervention to treat harmful conditions like *E. coli* infections and is also being considered as a cure for obesity.* Perhaps such research will find some tangible truth in the Three Worms theory and change the way that detox treatments are recommended.

In Taoist theory the Three Worms can divide and create Nine Worms, which cause exhaustion or sickness by blocking various points along the back. These worms have a bacterial or germlike nature and are linked to certain acupuncture points used to relieve their effects.

LOCATION OF THE NINE WORMS

ACUPUNCTURE POINT	ANATOMY	WORM TYPE
GV 16 feng fu	C1 Base of skull	Prostrating worm
UB 10 tian zhu	C1–2 (1.5 cun, or finger widths, lateral to midline)	Dragon worm
GV 13 tao dao	T1 (spinal process of)	White worm
GV 11 shen dao	T 5 (spinal process of)	Flesh worm

---

*For more on the gut biome see *The Diet Myth: The Real Science Behind What We Eat* by Tim Spector, which describes research undertaken by the British Gut Project at King's College London. Full bibliographic details are available in the recommended reading section.

LOCATION OF THE NINE WORMS (continued)

ACUPUNCTURE POINT	ANATOMY	WORM TYPE
GV 6 ji zhong	T11 (spinal process of)	Green worm
GV 5 xuan shu	L1 (spinal process of)	Worm of hindrance
GV 4 ming men	L2 (spinal process of)	Lung worm
GV 3 yang guan	L4 (spinal process of)	Stomach worm
GV 2 chang qiang	Tip of coccyx	Golden scale bug

PI GU REGIME IN THE DARKROOM RETREAT

As mentioned briefly in the previous chapter, the Pi Gu regime consists of a very specific diet of beverages and food, as well as our specially formulated elixir pill, although the exact components of the diet will vary somewhat from retreat to retreat.

Chlorophyll Drink

In the darkroom we drink a chlorophyll drink every day to clean out the blood and the large intestine. The chlorophyll drink cleanses and feeds on a cellular level, leading to health improvement.

Teas and Infusions

We have been serving what we call Immortal Tea in the Tao Garden restaurant for many years. This tea is one that Taoist masters have traditionally drunk. We also use this in the darkroom, as it increases urine production and is a good basic cleansing infusion for the kidneys and the liver. Immortal Tea is made from the *Gynostemma pentaphyllum* plant. Called Jiaogulan in traditional Chinese medicine, it has a reputation for increasing longevity, lowering cholesterol and blood pressure, and boosting the immune system. It is also a powerful antioxidant.

Mulberry leaf tea is regularly served in Tao Garden. Its natural benefits include blocking the body's absorption of some common sugars and containing vitamins and antioxidants. It strengthens the immune system as well as being useful for weight loss and diabetes management.

In the morning before breakfast, to help cleanse the lymphatic system and eliminate toxins in the liver, kidneys, and all other parts of the digestive system, darkroom participants take Native Legend Tea, a proprietary tea made up of five herbs: burdock, turkey rhubarb, sheep sorrel, slippery elm, and cress. This is followed by the antiparasitic tea mentioned above.

In the evening as a further detoxification for the digestive system plus the lungs, we serve Nature's T Infusion, a proprietary tea made up of nine herbs: senna leaf, buckthorn frang bark, peppermint leaf, uva ursi leaf, orange peel, rosehip fruit, marshmallow root, honeysuckle flowers, and chamomile flowers. It is sweet tasting and aids digestion. It, too, reduces cholesterol; it also reduces cellulite, and it helps to eliminate body odor by moving waste out of the body more quickly.

Pi Gu Elixir Pill

We have developed a Pi Gu pill, an elixir ball of herbs and fruit, which we serve twice a day during the darkroom sessions. Elixir pills are also used during the Pi Gu sessions that are part of the "Back to Body Wisdom" Taoist practices that Master Chia's teaches during his world tours.

Different Taoist schools would have had different versions of Pi Gu. Imagine the hermit or Taoist master wandering through the mountains, for many months or years. He would not be able to carry all of the food he would require with him and so to survive he would just eat some simple berries or nuts, together with water from the morning dew. Each Taoist sage would have his own secret formula of ingredients that he could pound together to create a supply of elixir pills, each one enough for a whole meal, ideal for carrying into caves.

We have developed our elixir pill, which we see as a great stimulus to the Pi Gu experience, based on a combination of many things mentioned in ancient texts (fig. 3.9). We commonly use a mixture of: Chinese plums or prunes, goji berries or other berries, walnuts, peanuts, black sesame seeds, herbs, pepper, hot spices, and dates, ground together and mixed with a little honey. The pills contain no sugar or additives. The exact composition of the elixir pills served at the darkroom retreats varies from year to year.

The instructions for eating the pill are as follows: Take it from its wrapping paper and breathe in its fragrance and sweetness before biting off a small part to chew. Chew very well and feel the saliva coming out. It is a meal in itself, and chewing it well facilitates the mixing in of a lot

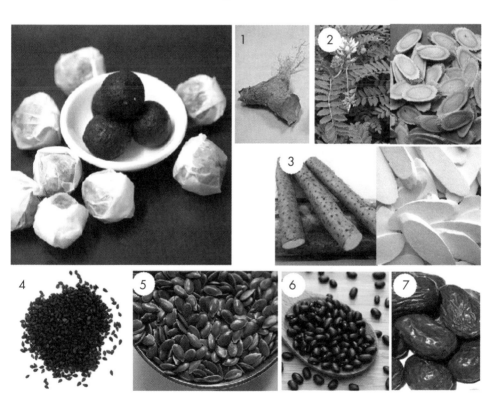

Fig. 3.9. Typical Pi Gu pill ingredients
1. Huang Jing (Solomon Seal) 2. Astragalus 3. Chinese yam
4. Black sesame 5. Flax seeds 6. Black beans 7. Chinese dates (Da Zao)

of saliva, sexual energy, hormones, oxygen, nitrogen, cosmic particles, and cosmic energy. The body will slowly create building blocks using the food and vitamins the body needs.

Pi Gu Food

The actual food we serve in addition to the beverages and the Pi Gu elixir pill is generally: steamed egg white, apple, pear, tomatoes, juju berries, goji berries, steamed peanuts, steamed edamame beans, and sesame. While detoxifying, excess fat goes into the waste system to be expelled and at the start of the process some participants suffer from typical detox symptoms such as headaches and dizziness. One way to avoid feeling weak is by keeping up a protein intake. That is why steamed egg white is included in the foods. This is a food that you chew very well and is also a building block for the body, which can be used for virtually anything needed. Vitamin C and fish oil are also added somewhere in the day's food to help in balancing the body's nutrients and cleansing.

TYPICAL DAY'S PI GU DIET IN THE DARKROOM

What follows is the basic outline of the Pi Gu diet as provided during the Tao Garden darkroom retreat. However, the exact makeup of the diet is not set in stone and will vary a little from retreat to retreat.

Drinks Taken throughout the Day

Native Legend Tea for lymphatic detox is drunk on rising or an hour before breakfast, along with (or mixed with) anti-parasitic teas, and often Jiaogulan (Immortal Tea).

There is a constant supply of ginger tea made daily from fresh ginger and water.

Mulberry leaf tea and a chlorophyll drink are served with lunch and Nature's T Infusion is served in the evening.

Before Breakfast

Red clover and possibly antiparasitic herbs in pill form, if not taken as a tea. The red clover combination capsules help to build the body's defense system and cleanse the tissues and cells. They can increase circulation and balance the glandular system.

Breakfast

One or two especially made Pi Gu elixir pills
Herb juice, which is also especially concocted
Steamed egg white
About twenty steamed peanuts or walnuts
One fruit: apple, pear, tomato, or goji berries

Lunch

Ginger tea or mulberry leaf tea (ginger tea is usually available
  at all times)
Chlorophyll drink (to cleanse the blood)
A thick sesame drink plus, or instead of, edamame beans
Fruit: watermelon pieces

Evening

One or two Pi Gu elixir pills (depending on individual
  energy level)
Fruit: apple, pear, goji berries, or juju berries
Nature's T Infusion sweetened with stevia plant

The evening infusion should be drunk before bed. It helps to clean out the bowels. In cases of constipation, the infusion should be left to soak for longer. Students can indicate to darkroom staff that they need the tea to be infused for longer if they feel the need. The body has twenty-six feet of intestines, so once they have been cleaned out, it will seem that they refill slowly; this could be mistaken for constipation. However, digestion will be much easier with this diet and the lack of toxins in the tubes. Participants will feel better and the food can move more quickly around the system. As we are eating less food, fiber can be added once daily to add more bulk to move out waste.

This regime might sound minimal, but in the darkroom there is an hour scheduled for eating each meal and a lot of this time is spent chewing. We are eating less than 50 percent of the usual amount but adding as much again in saliva by the extra chewing. It is the perfect opportunity to follow the Taoist maxim to the hilt: drink your foods and eat your liquids.

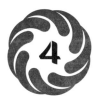

4

Chewing Chi Kung

The traditional Taoist saying "drink your food and eat your liquid" is one of the simple principles behind Pi Gu. We produce an average of a quart of saliva a day. It keeps the mouth and throat moist and helps the food go down to the stomach. It also helps activate blood. When it is sweet it protects tooth enamel. When it is sweet and fragrant, it has a longevity hormone in it; this flows out into the saliva when you are relaxed. However, when we eat hurriedly, we do not produce enough saliva. People's saliva is sometimes analyzed to determine their level of hormones; health issues can be diagnosed from seeing what gland secretions they may be lacking.

Saliva is a liquid, like water, and water is the most incredible solvent. Saliva is made up of 99.5 percent water. It also contains: mucus, electrolytes, glycoproteins, enzymes, and antibacterial compounds such as lysozyme and immunoglobulin A. The enzymes are very important, as they help to break down the food trapped in between teeth and are necessary to begin digesting starches and fats. Saliva can dissolve many things; indeed, the Tao says that saliva has ten times more power to dissolve than water. We can learn to chew the saliva for it to perform at its best as a transport system for distributing its essential enzymes, other ingredients, and oxygen around the whole body.

THE IMPORTANCE
OF CHEWING YOUR FOOD

Many cultures have maxims about chewing your food twenty, fifty, or a hundred times, but whatever the "correct" number, nowadays we do not chew enough. At mealtimes we consume many drinks, such as beer, wine, sodas, and juices while we eat. We eat a bit and drink a bit, alternating in a mechanical way, but the body does not like this, because the stomach does not receive the preorder for the right sort of gastric juices.

When we chew sufficiently, the saliva starts to flow and dissolves the aliments and oxygen from the air. The tongue tastes this mixture and informs the thalamus and hypothalamus, as the system can now detect what food is coming down. The stomach is thus prepared and knows what to expect. This is very important; otherwise it is like not booking the sort of hotel room you want and being disappointed at the reception desk. The glands—the thalamus and hypothalamus—are not warned, and this is made worse when you accompany the food with soft drinks or beer, drinking between mouthfuls of food and swallowing the food down quickly (fig. 4.1).

Even drinking a lot of water during mealtimes will dilute the gastric juices and the messages to the stomach. The stomach becomes confused and does not know what to do. The stomach's job at this point is to release the preordered digestive juices, and then to mix the juices with the food. But now it has to do extra work or digestion will not be achieved. Getting the right juices to come out takes a little time, and meanwhile, more food and beverages are on their way down.

One of the results of this style of eating is fermentation and gas. The stomach is like a bag that contracts and expands during its function. The perfect storm scenario is set up when you have a lot of gas: if the stomach is very distended by gas it cannot move in the way it should. Then further bloating occurs, and the food cannot mix with the juices.

At this point many people take indigestion medicine. However this

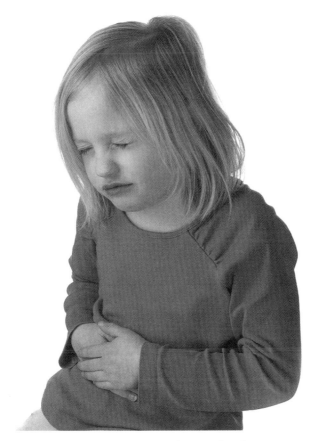

Fig. 4.1. Stomach is confused.

is usually alkaline to combat the stomach acid. These pills are generally 9–10 on the pH scale; some are even 14. But the stomach likes a balance of 7–8 pH and cannot work under these conditions. Thus the food is held in the stomach too long. That means that more acid is produced, with more gas as a consequence.

Pretty soon, the next meal will be on its way. Now the perfect storm has been whipped up: the stomach is in a state of distress; it has not finished one meal and has to cope with another one. When once again the stomach does not receive adequate warning about what digestive juices are needed, the problem is compounded. This can go on ad infinitum, or rather until there is a serious health issue in the stomach.

The overstressed stomach now pushes the problem further down the line into the small intestines. The stomach has not done its work and the small intestine cannot either. The food should be in very fine particles at this point, and if it is not, it cannot be absorbed into the walls of the small intestine through the villi (fig. 4.2).

There will likewise be a build up of problems in the small intestine. It will be taking much more time than it should to deal with the problem, so there is going to be some matter getting stuck in the system.

The food matter must be very small and well digested to be able to pass through the next part of the system, the ileocecal valve, which leads from the small intestines to the large one (see figs. 4.3 and 4.4 on page 62). If the food matter is not fine enough, a traffic jam is caused. The large intestine is there to get rid of the rest of the waste, but if the particles are not fine enough or there is any sort of build up, it will not be able to perform properly. One result will be the build up of toxins in the body. The nutrients and waste will take an excessively long time to go through the body. This is how sickness starts through toxins in the system. It will even bring on a feeling of tiredness or lethargy and affect mental, physical, and emotional well-being.

Taoist wisdom says "eat to fill your stomach two-thirds full" (see fig. 4.5 on page 63). This is simple to say but hard to follow, especially if you are partaking in a delicious meal or at an "all you can eat" outing. Other cultures have similar sayings. In Japanese it is *hara hachi bu*, meaning "eat until your stomach is 80 percent full." This is obviously easier in an Asian culture where food is served in smaller quantities than in the United States or parts of Europe. Using chopsticks to eat is also a way of putting less in your mouth than eating a hamburger held in your hand.

If you eat too fast, it will take some time for you to develop that sensation of "mmm, this is nice!" Then you get that feeling when you are already quite full and should really stop. But the "mmm, this is nice" feeling is going to incite you to have some more. Chewing better will

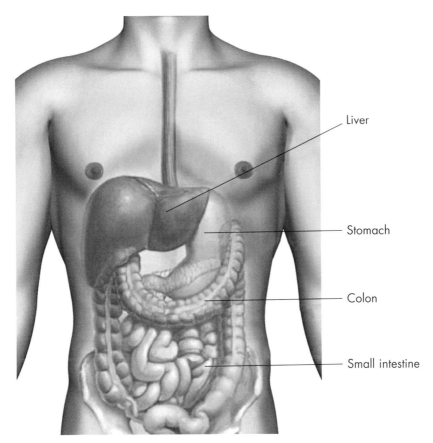

Liver

Stomach

Colon

Small intestine

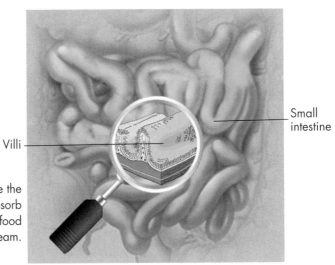

Small intestine

Villi

The villi that line the
small intestine absorb
small particles of food
into the bloodstream.

Fig. 4.2. Villi in the small intestine

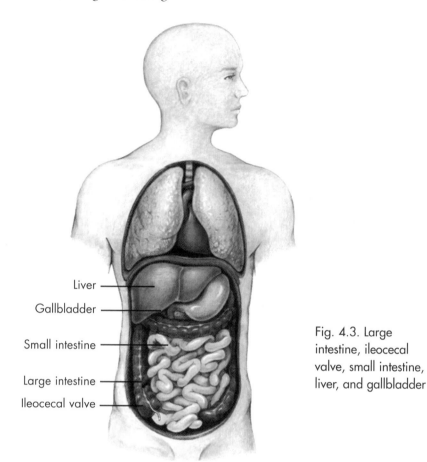

Liver

Gallbladder

Small intestine

Large intestine

Ileocecal valve

Fig. 4.3. Large intestine, ileocecal valve, small intestine, liver, and gallbladder

Ileocecal valve

Ileocecal valve

Fig. 4.4. Large intestine

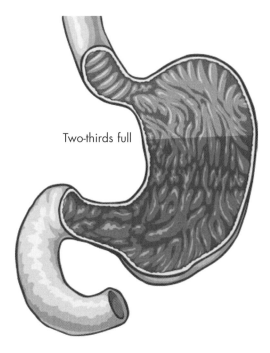

Two-thirds full

Fig. 4.5. Only eat to two-thirds full.

help you to stop before your stomach is full by inducing that feeling earlier.

Remembering a simple list of maxims will help you "eat your way to better health."

1. Chew a lot and produce saliva.
2. This preorders juices for the stomach.
3. Break down the food into small bits.
4. Do not swallow it until it is ready.
5. Drink sparingly during meals.
6. Stop eating before you feel full.

"EAT YOUR LIQUID"

In Pi Gu we do not just drink liquids down. First we mix them with saliva by taking a sip, then bending the head to one side and chewing the saliva. The chewing action produces saliva. Then we open the mouth wide and suck in air repeatedly to mix with it before we eat it; this is referred to as "eating the cosmos."

Imagine you are tasting wine (rather than actually drinking it): you swish it around your mouth, from side to side, moving it over all the taste bud areas in the mouth to release the flavors of the wine so that you can identify and analyze them. Treat each liquid in a similar way, and swallow it down only when you have mixed the saliva with the fluids. In this way the fluid mixture will be predigested. The body will know it does not have to do much with the mixture and let it go through the stomach faster.

When drinking Immortal Tea, for example, you can feel the sweetness of the tea. It is a natural product and you feel this against your tongue while the saliva is produced and mixes into it, and then you swallow it down hard and fast.

GETTING CHI BY CHEWING

As we have stated earlier, how we eat the food in Pi Gu is very important. If you just tried to stick to the food in the Pi Gu darkroom diet, it would not have any effect in itself, except that you would probably be hungry! But our darkroom participants do not feel hungry after meals. By looking at the quantity in the meals and comparing it in size to your "normal" diet, you can quickly see that there is a lot more to Pi Gu than lists of foods.

The most essential part of the Pi Gu mealtime is chewing, and the chewing is a form of Chi Kung in itself, as Chi Kung means "working chi." Pi Gu Chi Kung emphasizes two aspects of heightening chi through chewing. The first is that proper chewing allows us to absorb maximum chi from our food as we eat. The second is to draw in more chi from the universe when chewing.

When we are teaching Pi Gu practice we use certain foods—such as peanuts, walnuts, Chinese prunes, dates, and goji berries—as they are easy to chew, but need a lot of chewing, while at the same time are also simple to digest, with nutrients that we need. Taoist masters also chose these foods as they could easily find them in the rural places where they were living and meditating. Take care that the peanuts are still in their unpunctured shells so they are not contaminated or too dry. Similarly, it is important to choose Chinese prunes carefully, because if they are too dry then the seeds inside them will be very hard.

During the chewing, you must learn to listen to the chi and send it into your body through the ears. Ears have canals, and they go right into your nose, eyes, mouth, brain, and throat. Listen to this chi with a good mind, good heart, good chi, and let it flow into you.

When chewing, you are converting the food into a much more efficient energy by breaking it down with saliva and mixing in oxygen and nitrogen at the same time. If you chew well, you will also be able to take in cosmic energy (fig. 4.6).

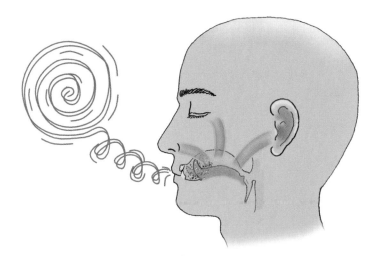

Fig. 4.6. Chew to blend saliva with Cosmic Chi.

Both the Bible and the Tao state that everything came from dust or cosmic particles, and they can therefore rebuild anything. As cosmic dust is what we are made up of, you can feel your saliva charged with Cosmic Chi turn into instant energy. But you need concentration and focus to get the energy. When chewing, draw in chi; then close your mouth so you can mix the energies. In this way the food acts as a medium for helping you to mix Cosmic Chi and saliva. They are mixed together into what Taoists refer to as "elixir." Why elixir? Because it can be converted into anything you need in your body.

EATING PEANUTS, WALNUTS, PINE NUTS—PI GU STYLE

We use peanuts in the Pi Gu practices in the darkroom because peanuts are one of the plants that fix nitrogen, via a bacteria that lives on their roots. They can convert this nitrogen into protein (fig. 4.7). Alfalfa also does this, along with other legumes (or dried beans). However peanuts can be eaten raw, whereas many legumes must be cooked for a long time and are eaten when soft or puree-like.

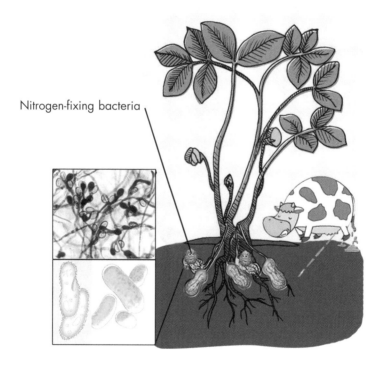

Nitrogen-fixing bacteria

Fig. 4.7. Peanuts fix nitrogen and are good to chew.

Some people don't like peanuts because of certain molds on them, but if they are dried and in a good intact shell, then there should not be any mold. In fact at Tao Garden we steam organically grown peanuts ourselves, although you can eat them raw. Obviously people with peanut allergies should use an alternative such as walnuts for chewing practice. Peanut allergies themselves are very complicated, so we cannot advise on whether some sources of peanuts could be safe for peanut allergy sufferers.

Chewing Saliva Chi Kung with Peanuts and Walnuts

This is not an exercise for a dinner party, as it can make a lot of noise, and it is rarely considered good etiquette to eat with your mouth open. However, it is inspiring to do this in a group, with everybody concentrating on the exercise, or just on your own. Focus on the chewing and feel a lot of saliva flowing into the mouth. Keep it all in your mouth and feel the mixture get bigger as the saliva increases and mixes into it.

1. Start by chewing 2–4 (according to their size) peanuts or walnuts (fig. 4.8).

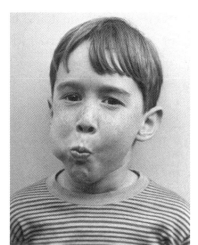

Fig. 4.8. Chew the nuts.

2. Do not swallow; chew continuously, varying the location from the left, middle, and the right sides of your mouth, as the saliva is different in different areas, which are attuned to different flavors (fig. 4.9).

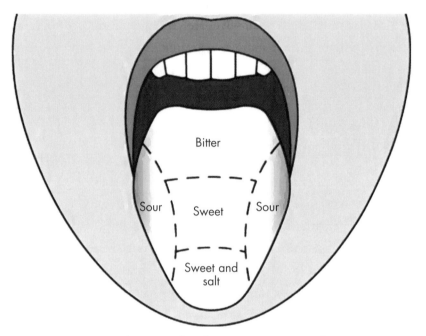

Fig. 4.9. The tongue has five main taste areas; these, in fact, represent the five elements.

3. Chew until there are no more lumps at all. If you don't chew well it can get stuck in the throat. The tongue is a great tool when chewing; use it to the maximum to move the food and saliva around. Different parts of the tongue are connected to different parts of the body. The tongue is the bud of the heart, which is connected with the element fire. Feel the heart fire connection as you chew (fig. 4.10).

4. Remember to relax, keeping the shoulders and the rest of the body loose, and smile as you chew. To help with doing this, remember what it was like to be a child. Children naturally start to chew with their mouths open, until they are taught not to eat that way.

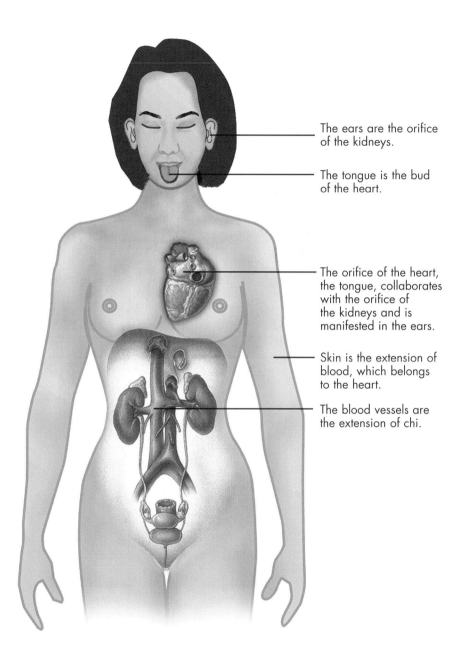

The ears are the orifice of the kidneys.

The tongue is the bud of the heart.

The orifice of the heart, the tongue, collaborates with the orifice of the kidneys and is manifested in the ears.

Skin is the extension of blood, which belongs to the heart.

The blood vessels are the extension of chi.

Fig. 4.10. Tongue connections

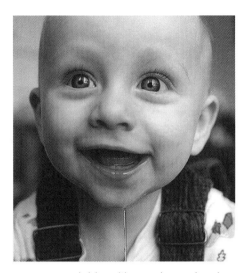

Fig. 4.11. Children like to play with saliva.

They also like to play with the saliva in their mouth (fig. 4.11).

5. As the saliva activates, you will become aware of your sexual organs.

6. Very gently breathing into your sexual organs, you will feel some kind of sexual energy come up.

7. You will feel the sexual energy go up to your glands, to stimulate them, and up to the brain to stimulate it.

8. As saliva increases, chew more, and more saliva will come out. At this point the peanuts are very liquid, thoroughly masticated, and dissolved in the saliva. Keep the liquid in your mouth.

9. Now rest, rub the hands together, and rub your nipples with them. This activates the thymus, parathyroid, thyroid, hypothalamus, thalamus, and pineal gland (the gland of light and of darkness).

10. There is even more saliva at this point. The way it is swallowed is important. Make your neck straight and swallow hard, sucking it in from the stomach.

11. Swallow like this 3 times and try to get it all down in those 3 swallows, being sure to keep the position of the neck straight (fig. 4.12).

12. Stroke your hands down the chest to help the chi go to the stomach (fig. 4.13).

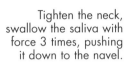

Tighten the neck, swallow the saliva with force 3 times, pushing it down to the navel.

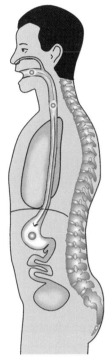

Fig. 4.12. Hold the neck straight and swallow 3 times to the stomach.

13. Keep your hands on your stomach and feel you are activating the original force.

14. Rub your navel and feel it become warm. Your stomach will feel

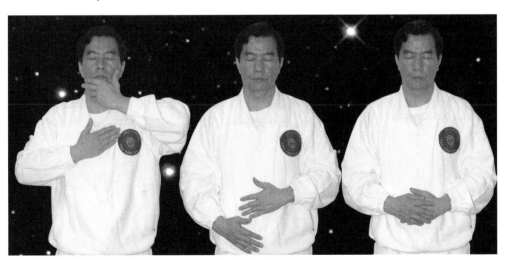

Fig. 4.13. Gradually bring the chi down to the navel.
Smile and feel the warmth.

warm, as your saliva plus oxygen, nitrogen, and chi is transforming into energy that is going to do whatever your body needs it to do. If you can get this feeling then you are starting to get the "Pi Gu effect." You might belch at this point.

15. Keep your hands on your navel, gently rubbing, as you feel the energy spread onto your hands and then down the legs; then rest (fig. 4.14).

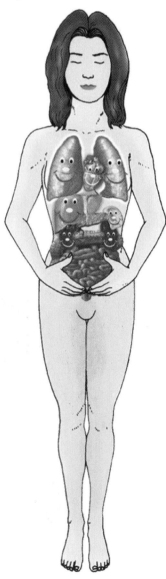

Fig. 4.14. Feel that smiling energy flow down into the organs and throughout the whole body.

The saliva that you have swallowed comes from several energies mixed together, but you are also using mind power to swallow. When you swallow, you must focus on the act of swallowing. You do not swallow as you would while eating a meal normally. You must swallow the peanut/saliva elixir both hard and fast, otherwise it will not go straight down to the stomach. From there the stomach will let it go down into the small intestine.

Avoid drinking anything, even water, at this point, so that the elixir mixture will stay in the stomach. We refer to it as elixir, as this saliva/peanut mixture has a lot of chi in it at this point. Adding drinks to this mixture will make it transit through the stomach more quickly, but because there is a lot of chi and dissolved nitrogen in the saliva that is beneficial for healing our stomachs, we want it to stay in the stomach longer to aid digestion.

Chewing Saliva Chi Kung Part 2

This Chi Kung is aimed at filling the stomach with chi, and this will lead us into a Chi Kung practice that shrinks the stomach. This exercise can be done without eating any food at the same time, just chewing to create saliva and working on the saliva—"eating the universe." Or it can be done while eating a small amount, as in the previous exercise, "Chewing Saliva Chi Kung with Peanuts and Walnuts."

1. Take a moment to be aware of your sexual energy, this can be helped by also doing Testicle or Ovarian Breathing (as detailed in our book *Basic Practices of the Universal Healing Tao,* pages 58–60 and 83–85; see "Recommended Reading" at the back of this book). When you do this for a while, energy goes up to the brain.

2. Activate your nipples, be aware of your glands: pituitary, parathyroid, thyroid, hypothalamus, thalamus, parathymus, thymus, and pineal. They are all connected to the saliva glands (see fig. 4.15 on page 74). As you chew and stimulate the sexual organs, sexual hormones

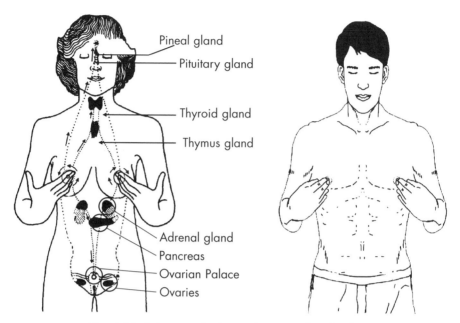

Pineal gland

Pituitary gland

Thyroid gland

Thymus gland

Adrenal gland

Pancreas

Ovarian Palace

Ovaries

Fig. 4.15. Rub your nipples and activate the glands.

come up and you start to receive chi from the universe. This attracts even more chi, which stimulates your hormone system. In this case it is the chewing that is the beginning of the cycle. You can also use the Nine Flowers Gland Massage (as detailed on page 35 of *Golden Elixir Chi Kung*) to mix the food and saliva with sexual hormones, with or without eating at the same time.

3. As you chew, keep your mouth partly open so air can enter and mix with the saliva (fig. 4.16). Chi will start to add itself to the mixture. As your teeth grind the saliva, focus on feeling that the food (if any), nitrogen from Cosmic Chi, and the hormone system are all mixing into this elixir together.

4. Even with the mouth shut you can feel chi coming into your mouth. Raise your hands out far, gather the chi, and inhale the Cosmic Chi, mixing it in with the saliva. Continue inhaling, feeling the noise in your throat. Repeat 1 more time, and continue chewing.

Be aware of the nature force, a beautiful mountain, a river, ocean, and beautiful flower garden. Extend your hands out to

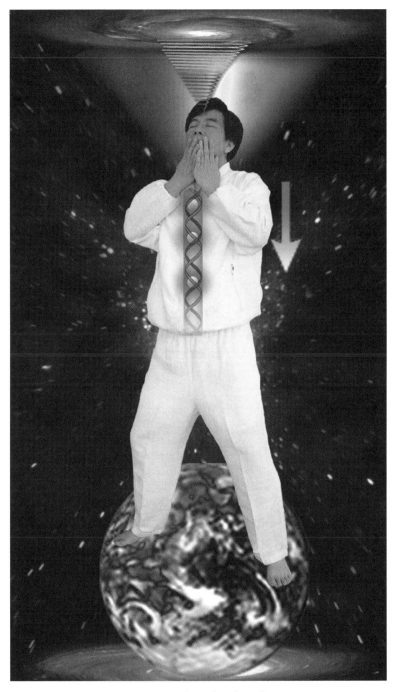

Fig. 4.16. Prepare the saliva by allowing air
to mix with it as you chew.

the universe. Open your palms and feel your arms and the palms grow very large and long as they reach out to nature and the universe (fig. 4.17). The original quantity of food is thus multiplied by ten.

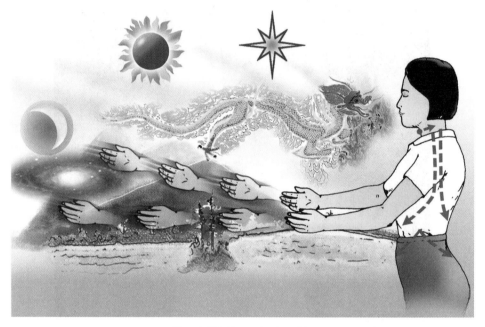

Fig. 4.17. Draw in the chi.

5. Now swallow down (as in the previous exercise): straighten the neck, helped by pushing the chin back and in (fig. 4.18). Swallow down the elixir hard and fast 3 times. This can be noisy and also cause you to belch.
6. Rub down with the hands from the chin to the stomach, while at the same time gently changing the weight from one foot to the other.

The Tao believes that if this elixir is well mixed, the stomach will have almost no work to do; digestion is much easier and "food" can be converted to energy very quickly.

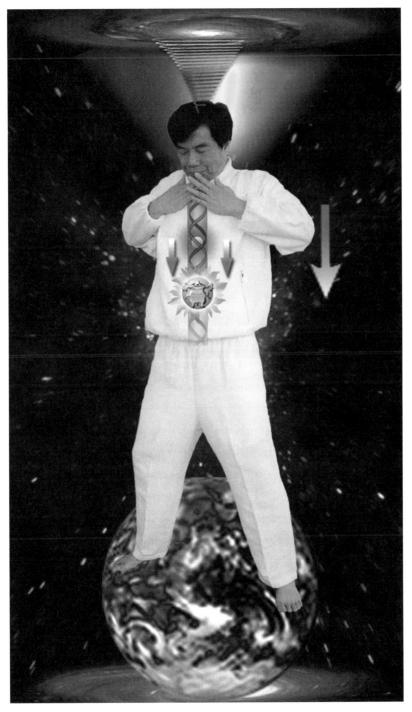

Fig. 4.18. Swallow the saliva down through chest, belly, and navel.

Chewing Chi Kung Part 3

Use this exercise to quiet the mind and temporarily let go of what you were doing before you started.

1. Take either an apple or a pear; one is enough for this exercise. Bite off a piece and just chew that piece, chewing it into small pieces, with saliva starting to flow so it sticks together.
2. Focus on the chewing, and relax. Eating when stressed, in a hurry, or thinking about too many things impedes saliva flow.
3. As more saliva comes, open your mouth, and continue chewing. As this is considered bad manners, this is better done alone or with other people practicing.
4. As you chew with your mouth open, feel the chi from the universe mixing in with your mouth contents. Think that you are absorbing the essences of nature—lakes, forests, and oceans—and the essences of the cosmos—clouds, cosmic particles, the sun, planets, and stars—and the universal essences—light, primordial force, and sacred spirit (fig. 4.19).
5. Everything in your mouth becomes a pulp. As it is liquid, you can rinse it around your mouth, going left and right.
6. Use the turtle throat position, as this activates the thyroid more (see fig. 4.20 on page 80). Focus on this activation, by visualizing your thyroid, as gland secretions flow into your saliva. Breathe into the throat, directly into the thyroid. Chi will be coming in.
7. Hands on navel, swallow the mouth liquid down hard 3 times. If it sticks in your throat it is because you have not chewed enough; it is a good test.
8. Rub the hands over the navel after swallowing and move your weight from one foot to the other, heel to toe.
9. Now rub the testicles or vagina area until you feel energy in the crown; hold the sexual area with one hand and with the other hand rub the tummy.

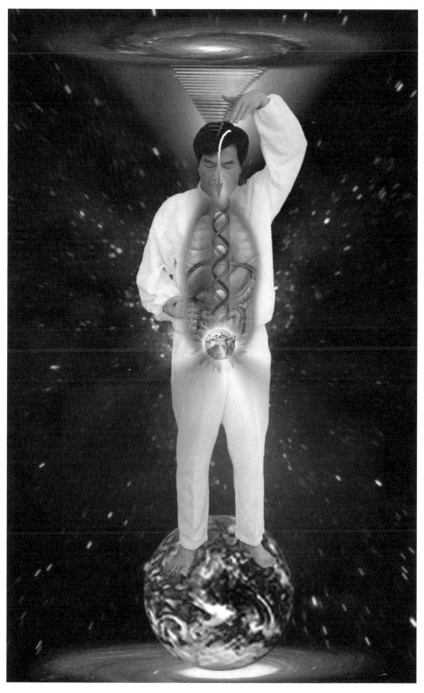

Fig. 4.19. Mix the energy of the earth, nature, and
the universe with the saliva in your mouth.

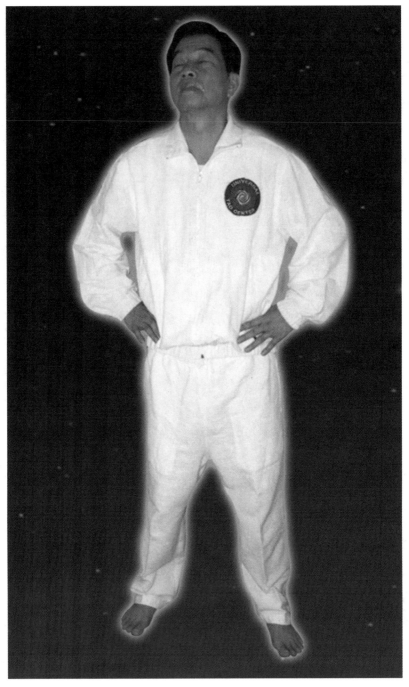

Fig. 4.20. Hold your neck like the turtle.

10. Feel the saliva mixing with the sexual energy and transforming into chi immediately.

   It is quite common to belch when you are rubbing the navel area, as the chi is moving in you. That is a good sign that the saliva you swallow down is transforming into chi immediately.

11. Change hands. As you continue rubbing, you will feel warmth in the abdomen; give your stomach the command to become smaller, to shrink. Do this every day and your stomach is going to get smaller.

Later on (in chapter 7, "Shrinking the Stomach") we will coordinate contractions in the other ring muscles—such as in the eye, perineum, and anus—with the ring muscle all around the stomach, to help heal it and reduce it in size.

Once you are familiar with the practices, as soon as you start chewing, you can go into practice mode. As you chew, focus on feeling the energy mixing with the food. The food becomes a medium for you, so chi goes to every part of your body through your mouth. When chi enters into your eyes, it goes to the mouth. You can smile as you look at trees and plants, and that chi is absorbed into your mouth. Expand your mind far away into the universe and you will absorb this chi into your mouth as well.

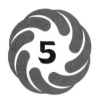

Basic Pi Gu Chi Kung

Some people try to achieve enlightenment at the cost of their bodies, but in the end they achieve neither good physical health nor enlightenment. That is why Pi Gu is so different as a form of fasting. Taoists believe that physical health aids spiritual development and enlightenment. Taoism aims to produce chi through the physical body in order to feed the souls and spirits for spiritual work. (See "The Five Enlightenments of the Tao" on page 23.)

By combining the Pi Gu fast (outlined in chapters 2 and 3) with greatly improved chewing techniques (given in chapter 4) and Pi Gu Chi Kung (detailed in this and the next two chapters), you can transform your body. We begin with some basic breathing exercises that are easy for the inexperienced. You might like to do these easier exercises several times before going on to the more advanced exercises given in the following chapters. You can also restart at the more advanced levels by summarizing the basic exercises prior to beginning or by remembering what it felt like to have the increase in chi from the previous Chi Kung.

Abdominal Breathing

Abdominal breathing helps you to breathe deeply, probably deeper than your normal breathing, by drawing the breath all the way down. It is energizing.

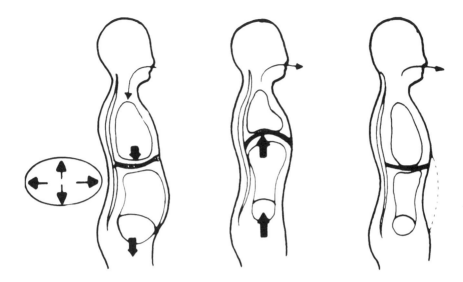

Fig. 5.1. Abdominal breathing

1. Breathe into the lower part of your abdomen, filling it as you breathe in, and emptying it as you breathe out (fig. 5.1).
2. While breathing in and out, place your hand on the lower part of the abdomen. This will help to focus your attention on the exercise and to remind you that you are filling the abdomen as you breathe in and emptying it as you breathe out; you will actually be feeling it under your hand.

Solar Plexus Breathing

The navel and the solar plexus area is where the stomach is located. We can learn to contract this area. It is both muscle and tendon together, a special sort of sack with sides like elastic bands. Like the stomach, it can expand and contract, like a strong plastic bag. Solar plexus breathing is just like abdominal breathing but a bit higher up.

1. Rub the solar plexus, and place your hand there; inhale into your hand and exhale (see fig. 5.2 on page 84).

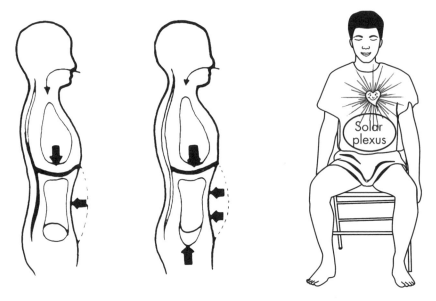

Fig. 5.2. Solar plexus breathing

2. Feel the saliva flow and focus on this elixir.

3. Inhale and exhale at least 30 times and then rest. When you do this, any trapped gas in the stomach will move down and out to the anus, which is the long way, or you will belch it up and out. Although belching sounds rude, it is a good sign. It shows that you are creating some space in your stomach.

Smiling to and Shrinking Your Stomach

After a certain age we do not grow upward, so we can only expand outward. On top of that, much of the food we eat today makes us spread out sideways. The body stores food for no reason. It does not know what to do with it, so it is laid down as fat cells. This exercise helps to shrink the stomach. Do not do this exercise on a full stomach; it must be at least partially empty. A good time is before lunch or other meals.

1. Smile to your stomach, feel your stomach, feel good chi (fig. 5.3).

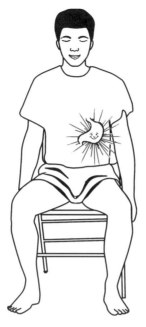

Fig. 5.3. Smile to your
stomach.

2. Now inhale, and when you exhale, feel that you are contracting
   your stomach. It is an involuntary muscle, so you cannot control it
   physically, but you can do so through your mind power, soul power,
   and subconscious.

3. Smile to your stomach, inhale, exhale, contract gently. Think
   of your stomach shrinking to its original size. See it happening
   (fig. 5.4).

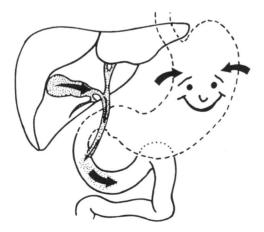

Fig. 5.4. Stomach smiling and shrinking

4. Rest and rub your stomach; you might belch, as when energy moves it usually pushes out a lot of gas. This resting phase of the exercise is very important. You have done some work, some Chi Kung, and now the body is using the chi; it is flowing around the body and making changes and healing.

Doing this Chi Kung in a group, with a Pi Gu–trained chi master, will help here. Master Chia passes energy to his students during these classes, helping them to give energy to their stomachs.

STIMULATING
THE DIGESTIVE SYSTEM

It is important that the digestive system work well and we can do some Chi Kung to improve it. This is particularly important if you fast, which is like shutting down a factory then finding it difficult to get it going properly again. In fact many big factories work day and night and do not even shut for holidays, because it is such a problem to get them going again. This hitting exercise strengthens the organs and increases the flow of the blood and chi.

This exercise is very good food for the digestive system itself; you are aiding the system to clear itself out so that food can pass on into the small intestines, whose function is to absorb nutrients. If the first part of the digestive system has worked efficiently, the small intestines' job will go more smoothly. Otherwise we will have a buildup of toxins in that part of the body, too, as there will be too many pieces of food that have not been predigested sufficiently. Valuable nutrients will not be in a condition to be absorbed by the small intestines and so will be lost to the body, going out as waste.

Taoists have done this exercise for a few thousand years, and we teach this as part of the morning exercise session at Tao Garden. It is also known as Stem Cell Chi Kung, as it stimulates stem cell production.

Digestive System Stimulation

Using a bamboo hitter, a hand, or other hitting tools, we are going to focus on our inner organs and hit them to release toxins (fig. 5.5).

We will be hitting the liver, gallbladder, stomach, spleen, pancreas, and small and large intestines. Your liver and gallbladder are on the right-hand side of your abdomen just below your ribcage. To the left is your stomach, then the spleen, and a little further down on the left-hand side is your pancreas. The small intestines are in the center of your abdomen below the stomach. And your large intestines encircle your small intestines.

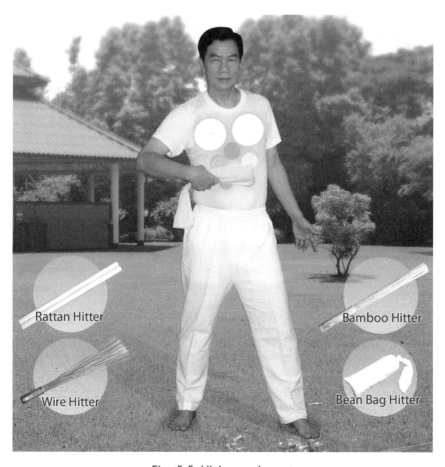

Fig. 5.5. Hitting equipment

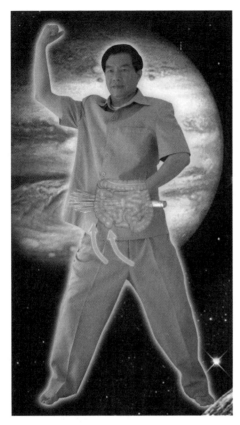

Fig. 5.6. Hitting stimulates digestive organ healing.

1. Stand with your knees slightly flexed, and rub the right-hand side of your abdomen below the ribcage to stimulate your liver and gallbladder. Then breathe into the area, hold your breath, and tap with the hitters at a steady rhythm (fig. 5.6).

2. Move to your abdomen just below the ribcage on the left to stimulate your spleen and stomach. Once again, rub the area you are working on, breathe into it, and hold your breath as you tap with the hitter. Then move down slightly to hit the pancreas. Stimulating these organs will probably make you belch, releasing trapped gases in the digestive system.

3. Repeat: Liver, gallbladder, spleen, stomach; then go down a bit to hit the pancreas. Rest for a little while to allow the chi and blood to flow through these organs. Then warm up the organs by rubbing the surface of the body.

4. Stimulate the stomach and intestines on the interior left: Inhale and pull up, spiral, pack, and squeeze energy into the interior left abdominal line (fig. 5.7). This channel runs parallel to the center line, vertically between the ribs and the pubic bone, one and a half inches to the left of the navel. While maintaining the pressure, hit down to the pubic bone and then back up the same line to a point just below the rib cage. Exhale, relax, and absorb the chi.

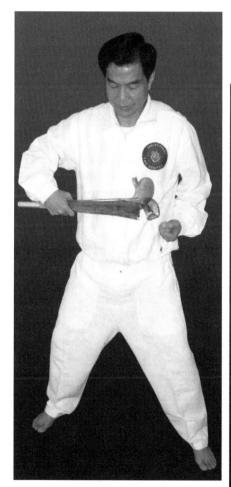
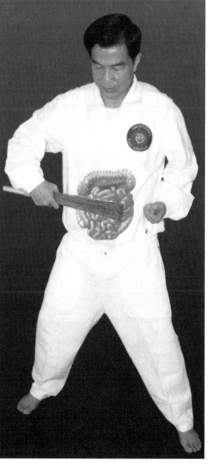

Fig. 5.7. Hit the stomach and intestines on the interior left abdominal line.

5. Move a few inches to the left and repeat step 4 on the exterior left abdominal line.

6. Now hit the interior and exterior lines on the right side of the abdomen using the same procedure as in steps 4 and 5 above. Use the left hand to hit as the right hand covers the right kidney, or remains in a fist (fig. 5.8).

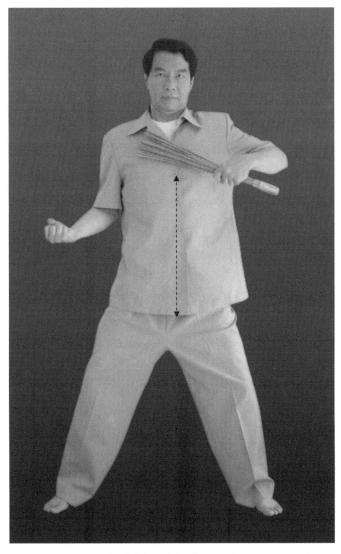

Fig. 5.8. Use the left hand for hitting the interior and exterior lines on the right side.

7. Stimulate the small intestine: First, rub around it in a circle. Feel the gut being activated, the blood flowing more freely, and the pockets of trapped gas being released. Breathe into the area, hold the breath, and start hitting from top to bottom.

   Do not forget the rest period; rub the whole area and feel good, particularly in the small intestines, feeling they can absorb the nutrients and eliminate the waste.

8. Now move on to the large intestine. First shake the colon with your hand and make it move to stimulate release of matter stuck to the walls. Start with the ascending colon on the lower right-hand side of your abdomen; move up to the transverse colon, which crosses your abdomen from right to left, and then move down the descending colon and sigmoid colon on the left-hand side of your abdomen (fig. 5.9).

   Now tap the colon with your fist in the sequence outlined above.

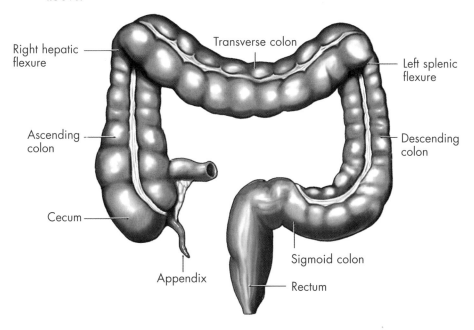

Fig. 5.9. Hit the large intestine, moving up the ascending colon, across the transverse colon, and down the descending colon.

Note: Always hit or massage in this direction, which is the natural direction of waste elimination, to encourage stuck waste matter to flow from intestines to rectum to anus. Never use the reverse direction.

It is very important to keep the digestive system working; the chi it produces is what keeps everything going. Refine this chi to create a link between the body, the soul, and the spirit. When the chi is more refined we call it *shen,* which is the food for the soul and the spirit. That is one of many reasons that Chi Kung is so important in Pi Gu.

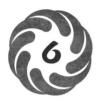

Harmonizing Chi with Alignment Chi Kung

THE IMPORTANCE OF CHI KUNG IN PI GU

Chi Kung is an important and effective means to work on your chi to achieve Pi Gu effects. We must use the energy around us, but when your own chi is not aligned properly, you cannot use it. When your own energy—the energy inside of you—is good, you can positively affect the energy around you by aligning it with your energy (fig. 6.1).

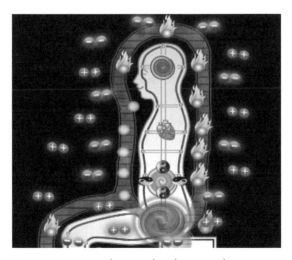

Fig. 6.1. Aligning the chi around us

This Chi Kung works by converting outside energy into usable energy for your body. The theory is that when you have abundant chi in the body, then it no longer needs to take in external energy as food. With the Pi Gu practice, the body has started to learn how to convert energy from outside to nourish itself. When you have reached this point of obtaining your nourishment from chi, you will feel full and stop eating. When you start eating again your body will have changed, reset itself. Your diet desires will have changed, and your diet will continue to modify each time you go through a Pi Gu experience long enough to achieve this.

We say that chi makes chi. A person who has weak chi because of being overweight/underweight/or otherwise in poor body health cannot make much chi. On the other hand, we have all met people who can make a whole room feel good as they naturally, or through meditation work, make the chi around them positive. Eating healthily will help your chi, and a mindset of love, joy, and happiness will ensure that your chi is properly aligned. Then your mind-heart-soul power can change the chi outside.

PRACTICING ALIGNMENT
AND DIRECTING CHI INTO YOUR BODY

We do this Chi Kung standing up, as in many moving forms of Chi Kung and also Tai Chi. If you can feel the chi aligned in this form, then any Tai Chi or Chi Kung that you do will be effective. Sometimes there are too many movements in a long Tai Chi form and it is difficult to feel chi; if you cannot feel the good energy and realign the energy outside of you, then you cannot use such long Chi Kung forms.

When you have good chi you do not need more movements; you just have to get one movement right and you can feel the chi, harmonize it, and integrate it. This good chi inside means that you can affect the chi outside.

Begin with a Smile

The simple part to understand is: if you have good mind and a good heart, you will then have good chi.

1. To practice this simple mindfulness, think "good, joy." Be happy, think happy, feel loving chi, smile down to the lower tan tien with your good mind and good heart, and you will have good chi flow.
2. Be aware of the universe above you, below you, in front and behind, all spiraling (fig. 6.2).

Feel the universe charge your lower tan tien and the tan tien charge your heart and small intestine.

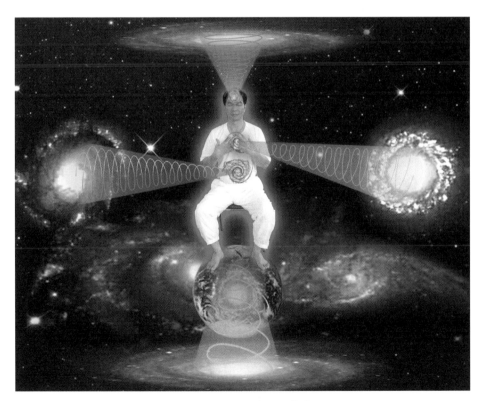

Fig. 6.2. Energy comes from all directions.

Alignment Chi Kung Part 1

When energy is not aligned properly, you cannot use it. Understand the difference between the energy inside your body and the energy that is outside your body, in the air around you. When your own energy is good you can positively affect the energy around you by aligning it with your energy. Practice aligning the chi in this way; otherwise the energy inside stays the energy inside and the energy outside stays the energy outside, and they are not connected.

1. Very slowly put out your hands, palms downward. Very slowly feel your chi through your palms. We are quite used to feeling our fingers and hands, but less so our palms.
2. Breathe in, breathe out, and feel something tingling through your palms. When you feel your palms have good energy, you can convert the energy to become electron negative-positive aligned.
3. Slowly move your palms; feel relaxed while moving the palms slowly. Now start to use your mind to talk to the energy outside. Tell it to align, to become good energy, so that you are surrounded by good energy (fig. 6.3).

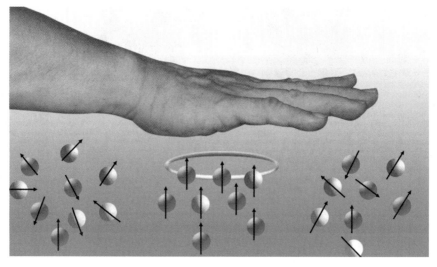

Fig. 6.3. Your hand aligns the chi outside.

4. Bring your hands up, slowly; you should have no appointments, no planes or trains to catch during a meditation, so do not hurry. Focus on feeling the energy follow you as you slowly move your hands up and down. Inhale as you move your hands up, feel the chi inside too, focus on your good chi, good mind, and good heart. The energy will start to align (fig. 6.4).

5. We are now ready to expand the chi; we can go to many different levels. There is a different chi at each level. First you align with the

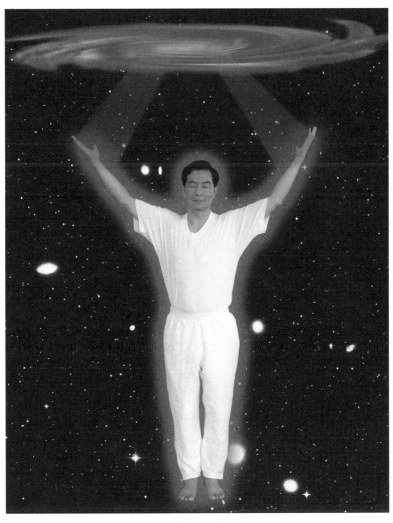

Fig. 6.4. Aligning the energy

cosmic particles, then with Primordial Chi, and then with the creator. All the levels have different energies but at this moment we want to get in touch with the energy around us.

Spiral your hands and you are spiraling the chi, very slowly. Smile; feel the chi is following you (fig. 6.5). The energy outside is very similar to the energy inside you now.

6. Sink down a bit, gather the chi, and condense the chi from the outside, pushing it into the lower tan tien. Feel the chi stay with you and command it to stay.

7. Inhale, come up very slowly—there is no hurry, remember "no appointments." Exhale, expand the chi and your mind very far away.

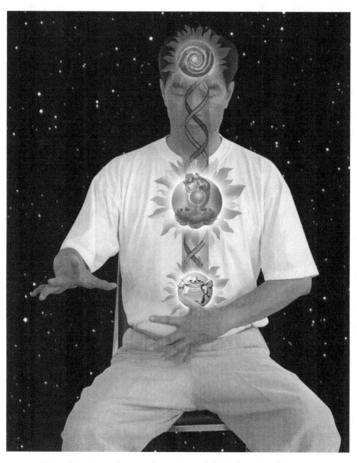

Fig. 6.5. Spiral your hands and feel the chi change.

8. Spiral with your palms, breathe in and breathe out, and condense the chi. Feel the chi outside of you as it starts to become your own chi inside. Condense this chi inside and it will now be the same energy as the chi already inside of you.

9. Inhale and focus on feeling the earth force coming up and expanding out to the universe (fig. 6.6).

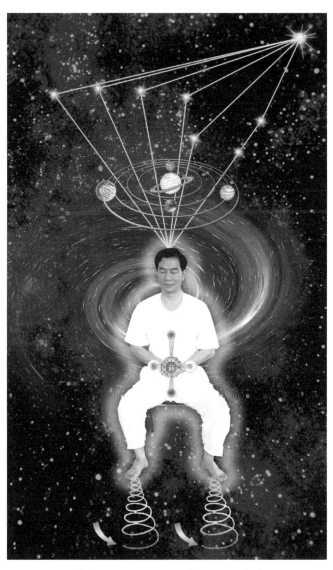

Fig. 6.6. Earth force comes up and mixes with the universe.

10. Smile; expand your good chi, good heart, good mind; and spiral. Exhale, condensing the chi. While breathing slowly and smiling, feel yourself holding this chi for 5 minutes.

11. Once again, inhale, feel the chi follow you; exhale, spiral, bring in the chi. Now it is aligned and similar to your own energy. Condense the chi, hold the chi, put the tip of your tongue up to touch behind your upper teeth (fig. 6.7).

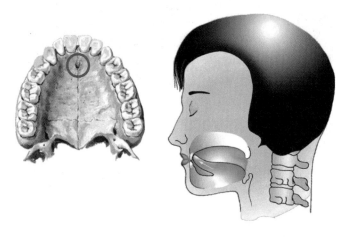

Fig. 6.7. Touch your tongue to the roof of
the mouth to make the connection.

12. Feel relaxed; when the chi circulates, it will activate your elixir—your saliva. More saliva flows and it becomes sweeter and more fragrant as the chi flows.

13. Expand the chi; fill up your stomach and small intestines. Chi, as nutrient fuel, is the end product of food ingredients; however, if you can convert this chi from outside then you need less food. Alignment Chi Kung trains the body to do this conversion.

Alignment Chi Kung Part 2

After the first part of the Chi Kung you will have good energy. This is the energy that you need to convert to chi in your body.

1. Hands on the sides, feel the chi. Continue to move it very slowly in small spirals. Condense the chi around you and put it into your chi. Feel this powerful chi as you condense all the chi into one chi and direct it right into the top of the head.

2. Feel the very condensed chi flowing right into your crown (fig. 6.8). Breathe in, breathe out, and focus on putting more chi right into your brain, then penetrating into the middle of your body all the way down to the perineum.

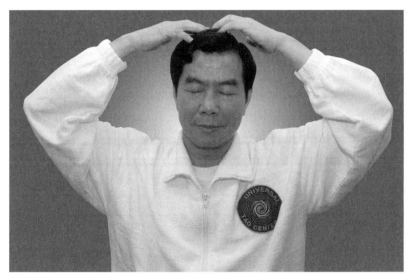

Fig. 6.8. Chi flows into the crown of the head.

3. Inhale, then exhale with your tongue up. The more chi you get, the more elixir will flow as the chi stimulates the glands and the saliva system. As your saliva increases with gland secretions, more elixir will nourish your system. The entire hormone system, the glands included, can take in more energy than other body cells.

4. Feel chi go right into the crown and down to the perineum; feel chi open its passageway so your body can take it in more easily. This is Pi Gu Chi; it is fundamentally important to understand this energy opening in Pi Gu practice and also important to feel it happening. If you cannot get this part then you cannot get the Pi Gu effect.

☉ Two Beaks

Now we are going to use two beaks, from the Tai Chi form. The beak is used because it has a lot of power inside of it and we can channel the power through the point. Here we are going to use the beak to send energy to the ears, as they are connected to the eyes and the brain and, in fact, everything.

1. Inhale, smile, think: good chi, good mind, good heart, love, joy, happiness. Let the good chi combine with the mind and heart and let this good chi radiate out.
2. Move your arms very slowly and feel the chi follow you. The more you train the more you can convert this chi and use it. When you are ready with the chi that you gather in the hand, put the pinky fingers in the middle with all the other fingers pressing on the pinky to form a beak (fig. 6.9).

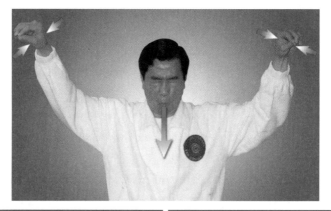

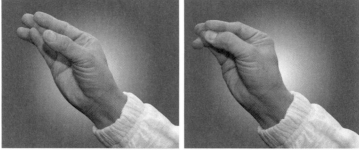

Fig. 6.9. Move your arms to gather chi, then form the beak.

3. Inhale, form the beak with your fingers, and gather the chi as you do so. Exhale, pushing the chi right into the ears. Breathe in, breathe out, and on the exhale, project the spiraling chi right into the ears through the beak. Send it spiraling round the ear, then down the external auditory ear canal.

4. Again inhale, exhale, and project chi. Feel the chi go into the ear canal, into the eyes, into your brain, and go right into your organs. In this way your body will start to receive this more direct chi; your organs and your body start to learn what it feels like and how to receive energy directly in this way. Again inhale, exhale, put chi right into your ears, and do this for about 3 minutes.

5. Smile and lightly turn up the corners of the mouth. Feel the chin bones on both sides rise up and reach to the ears, and feel the ears getting longer and longer, growing up and down and reaching the kidneys and other organs (fig. 6.10).

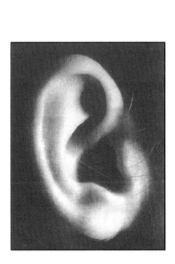
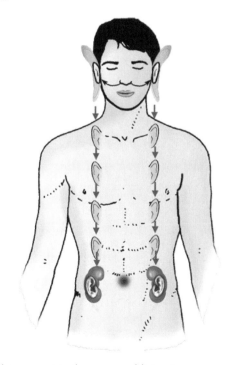

Fig. 6.10. Smile and feel chi connect to the ears and listen to the kidneys and other organs.

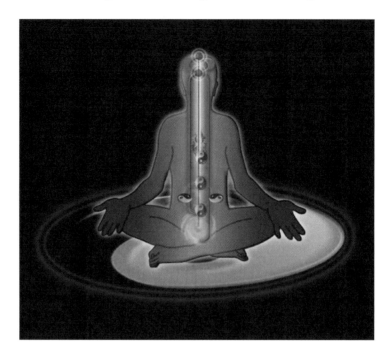

Fig. 6.11. Energy flows down from the crown.

6. Sit down and feel the energy flow in the open crown and down (fig. 6.11).

Reviewing the exercise, we can say that it is very simple:
1. You have to think that you have good chi.
2. You are capable of affecting the chi around you.
3. Your crown is open so that you can take the chi in directly.

If you practice this alignment, then when you do Tai Chi or Chi Kung you can apply it and feel the effect.

AVOIDING KUNDALINI PSYCHOSIS

Occasionally people who have experimented with certain meditations end up suffering from what we call the "kundalini psychosis" or "kundalini syndrome." It is a sort of Cosmic Chi indigestion, arising when the central channel was opened from the crown, usually by another person, and energy poured in, but the receiver was not yet ready to do the visualization work of controlling the energy for himself or herself. As a result, the chi could not be digested, as it was not converted in the proper way. Prematurely opening the kundalini channel in this way can result in a variety of physical and mental effects ranging from oversensitivity to touch, light, and sound to emotional dysregulation to symptoms such as head pressure, pain around the heart, and shaking, tingling, or pulsating sensations. "Opening the Kundalini" for another person is not a Taoist practice. But learning to align the chi as described above in Alignment Chi Kung will help you to avoid the problems associated with premature opening described here.

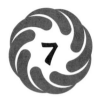

Shrinking the Stomach

We have seen that the stomach can expand to five times its original size. Looking at morbidly obese people, we might think that it can actually expand even more than that! Once the stomach has expanded, it requires more food to fill it. In fact, the appetite will have expanded too. It is very difficult to reduce the stomach size once it has expanded; it is like a deflated balloon that cannot keep its original elasticity, especially if it has been overstretched for a long time. As a result, stomach reduction surgery is a growing market in medicine. But instead we need to make the stomach feel its elasticity again. Taoists have a Chi Kung for doing this too.

This Chi Kung will help you to reset your body wisdom. The stomach is the place where all the food you eat is converted into energy, so if the stomach is not good and happy, you will not be able to get enough good nutrition. Therefore the first thing you need is your mindset, then a good variety of food. Next, if you chew well, you will double this effect. Cut down the food by at least 10 percent; this is a mechanical necessity to give the stomach room to work better and start healing (fig. 7.1).

This Chi Kung will help you to shrink the stomach and regain its elasticity. Then it will be easier to get in touch with the sensation of the stomach being happy before it is filled with too much. You must

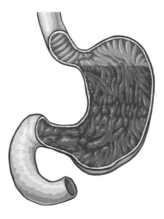

Fig. 7.1. The stomach needs some empty space in it to work properly.

learn to recognize the point where the taste may still be good but the stomach needs you to stop eating. If you get your full appetite back and start to eat too much again, then go back to doing the exercises.

RING MUSCLE MEDITATION AND CHI KUNG

The stomach is a ring muscle, or a sphincter muscle, which is a round muscle around an orifice. The word *sphincter* is generally associated with the anus, so we will use *ring muscle* as the general term for this type of muscle. A ring muscle is a special tendon/ligament structure with blood vessels in it. The ring muscles in the body are: the uterus, the muscles around the eyes, the urinary canal, certain mouth muscles, the anus, and the stomach. These muscles work as a team in the body: they have a connection with each other and with the rest of the systems of the body (see fig. 7.2 on page 108). When the heart pumps blood into the ring muscles, they all, including the stomach, which is the largest ring muscle, contract and expand.

Our eyes are very important in Ring Muscle Chi Kung, as we can contract the eye muscles voluntarily; that is, by ourselves. The connection of the eyes to the stomach goes beyond that highlighted by the expression for a greedy child who serves himself too much to eat: "his eyes are bigger than his stomach." When contracting the muscles around

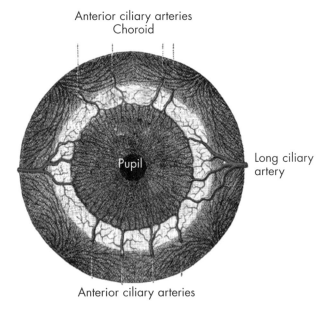

The sphincter muscles in the face connect to the anal sphincter and the sexual sphincter muscle.

External urinary sphincter anal sphincter muscles of female

External anal sphincter muscle of male

Fig. 7.2. All the ring muscles are connected and work as a team.

the eyes, the iris expands and contracts and it influences the involuntary muscles of the ring muscles circle (fig. 7.3). Each ring muscle "tickles" the other muscles, making them all want to contract together. Your mind can think your stomach smaller when accompanied by Chi Kung in this way.

Anterior ciliary arteries
Choroid

Pupil

Long ciliary artery

Anterior ciliary arteries

Fig. 7.3. Eye muscles work with our other ring muscles.

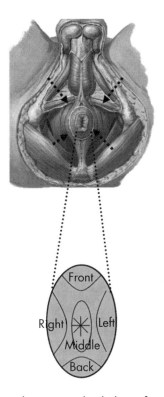

Fig. 7.4. The anus is divided into five parts.

The anus is important too as we can control the contractions of this sphincter (fig. 7.4). In fact there are many Taoist practices that involve contracting the anus muscles. (See *Tan Tien Chi Kung* for more information.)

There are also nonring muscles that work with the ring muscles: in the eyebrows and eyeballs, as well as the nostrils, tongue, and ears. They are coordinated with the hands and feet. The ring muscles are also connected to the blood vessel network, which becomes the largest honorary member of the ring muscle team.

The ring muscles are connected to the digestive system and also the breathing system; in fact, all body functions feel their influences. When the stomach is in the poor distended state described above, its imbalance will affect the other ring muscles and the general health of the body. So getting your stomach back in shape will be good for your whole body too. The amazing thing that ancient Taoists discovered is that the other members of the "ring muscles team" can help to correct it and get it back into shape.

The Ring Muscle Chi Kung exercises help you learn how to gather chi and then direct where you want it to go with your mind. You can keep that good energy state and feeling through doing these meditations and Chi Kung.

Ring Muscle Chi Kung Part 1

1. Smile, rub your stomach, and keep your hand on your stomach, so that you can feel your stomach contract and release under it.
2. Start with the anus, contracting it gently, and you will start to feel the stomach contract; let go and feel the stomach release gently, then contract again; feel the elasticity of the stomach.
3. Relax and you will feel warm as you gather chi slowly by contracting the eyes and the anus at the same time.
4. Keep your focus on your stomach contraction. Even if you feel the brain contracting too, leave that in the background.
5. Place the tip of the tongue behind the upper teeth.
6. Just take the mind to the good energy contracting the stomach; inhale, exhale, and contract.

Go Back to the Feeling

Once you have taken time to do these practices and set up your proper energy pattern, you can go back to that feeling. You will then need a shorter time to do the practices in the future. When you have some empty time, you can just spiral, feeling so nice and good in the stomach (fig. 7.5).

Ring Muscle Chi Kung Part 2

The stomach works all the time when there is food in it. When the stomach loses elasticity, heal it by using other ring muscles, mainly the

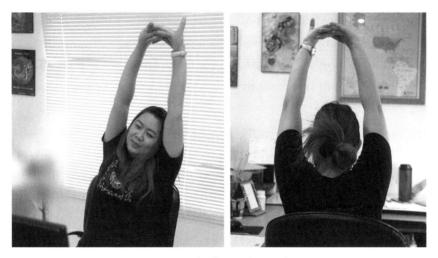

Fig. 7.5. Use your ring muscle discreetly in otherwise empty time.

perineum, anus, mouth, and eyes. You cannot do this exercise if the stomach is full. So choose a right moment.

1. Contract the eyes gently, not straining, and the stomach will follow the example and contract. Suck your eyes into the sockets and into the crown (fig. 7.6).
2. Draw the ears toward the ear canals and to the mouth.

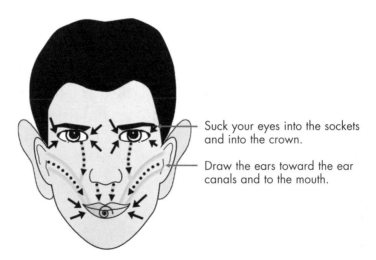

Suck your eyes into the sockets and into the crown.

Draw the ears toward the ear canals and to the mouth.

Fig. 7.6. Contract the eyes and draw the ears to the mouth.

3. Begin to do gentle anus contractions; since your stomach will follow by contracting, you might belch to expulse gas. The anus triggers the other ring muscles into contracting. Then you will feel something inside of you contracting; you will be aware of your stomach contracting.

4. Keep in mind that the stomach is getting smaller and feel its elasticity.

5. Focus on the stomach, even though you might feel the brain contracting too.

6. Put the tip of the tongue up to the roof of the mouth behind the upper teeth and saliva will start to come.

7. Rest after 5 minutes and feel the stomach; it should feel warm and good. When the human body is exercised in the right way, it will respond in the right way.

8. Continue the gentle contractions for another 4 minutes. Just feel you have good chi, and love, joy, and happiness.

9. Let it radiate out in your body and let it affect the chi around you; continue to feel the stomach warm inside you and under your palms.

10. Now move the hands slowly up and down, and the chi will feel sticky around you. Stroke down the body to prevent the chi from sticking, first with one hand, then with the other hand, then with both at the same time (fig. 7.7).

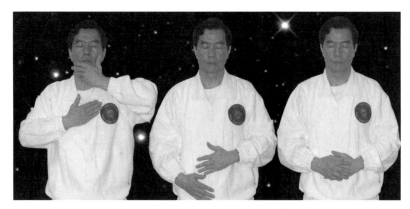

Fig. 7.7. Stroke down the body to prevent the chi from sticking, first with one hand then with the other hand, then with both at the same time.

11. Spiral slowly. Feel the energy around you align and stick to your hands and skin.

12. Gently breathe in and feel you are breathing in the chi.

13. Exhale, condense the chi. Spiral with the hand slowly, feel warmth and happiness in your joints, let the love and joy radiate out to your whole body.

14. Feel the stomach warm. With the sacrum tucked in, inhale, press from the sacrum to roll the body up, condensing the chi into you. Move the sacrum up again, drop your lumbar, round your back, inhale, roll your body upward, exhale, and condense the chi.

15. Hold your stomach and think of it contracting, getting smaller; feel its elasticity becoming more vital.

16. Smile to your perineum and relax.

17. Give the command to your stomach: "small"; will it to become smaller; there is no need to have a big stomach.

18. Focus on the chi and give it the command "small."

19. Gently contract the eyes, make them very gentle; feel the connection to the stomach as the stomach also contracts.

20. Remember this good feeling and program it to stay in you.

21. Look for that feeling when you have eaten enough to feel satisfaction and have chewed enough to satisfy the brain and hypothalamus.

22. When you feel this, multiply that feeling to the whole body (see fig. 7.8 on page 114). When you feel that your stomach is contracting and expanding, then this is the moment that you can copy the feeling. Concentrate and copy it and then start the movement again.

23. Relax, cover your stomach, and just smile to it.

24. Feel it nice and warm and feeling good; you now know the difference between an upset stomach, which does not feel good, and this stomach you have made feel good.

25. Rub the stomach clockwise, condensing in the energy.

You must learn to expand this good feeling. Let the body remember it and want to achieve it again. When you shrink your stomach down,

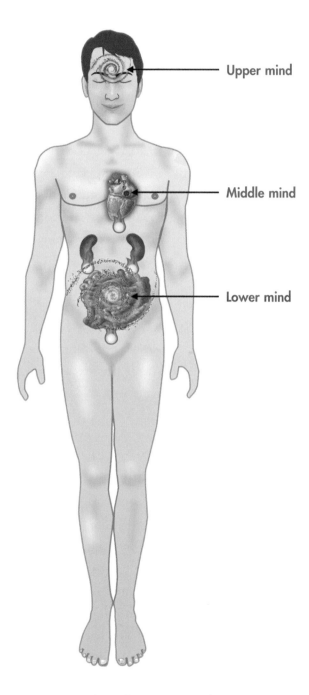

Fig. 7.8. Feel good in your stomach.
Relax and smile down—copy the feeling.

you will need less to fill it, and that will continue as you reduce the overall quantity of food you eat. Try this for a month, expanding the feelings of fullness. Eat 50 percent less and you will feel good. But when you eat more than 70 to 80 percent again you will not feel so good. So try eating 50 percent again and you will then feel that is satisfactory. You will remember this feeling.

When teaching Pi Gu, Master Chia sends energy to help the students, particularly during these stomach contracting exercises. After training with him you can go back to the exercises at any time, even for five minutes, to regain this feeling.

Golden Elixir Chi Kung

Taoists have given the name Golden Elixir to the mixture of saliva fortified with hormones and chi, which is seen as a complete nourishment with healing properties. Golden Elixir aids transformations in Inner Alchemy spiritual practices; that is why it is so important in Pi Gu. If you are trying Pi Gu to lose weight or reset your body metabolism, it can also play a very powerful role in these processes.

We will be working with the endocrine system in this section, using the power of the glands. The hypothalamus produces a protein, POMC, which limits appetite and food intake; it causes people to feel full and stop eating. Scientists at Yale School of Medicine are researching ways to use this knowledge for our benefit, but Golden Elixir Chi Kung will already improve your gland health.

Golden Elixir Chi Kung Part 1

This Chi Kung is for both men and women.

1. Rub the hands together and cover the breasts for a moment to feel chi.
2. Feel the chi on your breasts; touch the nipples and spiral in little

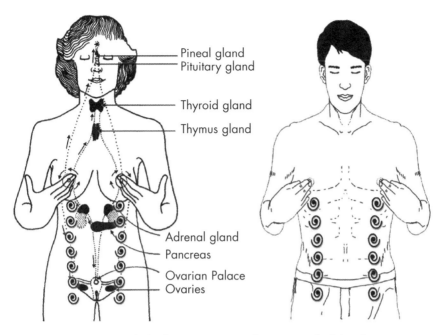

Pineal gland
Pituitary gland

Thyroid gland

Thymus gland

Adrenal gland
Pancreas

Ovarian Palace
Ovaries

Fig. 8.1. Rub the breasts in a circular motion; feel the chi
as you spiral it down the nine flowers.

circles. Expand your mind, feeling your nipples and feeling the connection of chi in the thymus gland in the chest (fig. 8.1).

3. Spiraling with the fingers, let the chi go into the thymus, and then
   throughout the endocrine system, going into the pineal gland, pituitary gland, thyroid gland, para thyroid, adrenal glands, pancreas,
   ovarian palace, ovaries or testicles. Imagine that you have "nine
   flowers" or energy nipples extending down the front of your body.

4. Let the chi flow into your throat center, thyroid, and parathyroid;
   wrapping the energy around the glands, feel the sensation.

5. Visualize your pituitary gland, positioned at the base of the brain,
   almost midway on the line between the mid-eyebrow and the back
   of the head (see fig. 8.2 on page 118).

6. Be aware of the spiraling energy going up to the thalamus and hypothalamus; feel the connection.

7. Tap the top of the crown above the pineal gland, know where it is
   located, and guide chi from the nipples to the pineal gland.

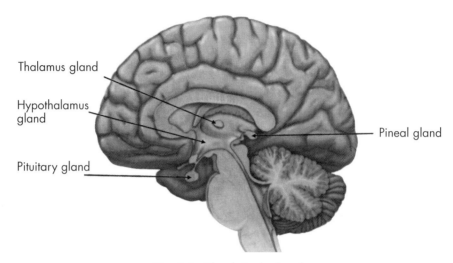

Thalamus gland

Hypothalamus gland

Pituitary gland

Pineal gland

Fig. 8.2. Glands in the head

8. Visualize the adrenal glands about 2 inches above the navel at the back of the abdomen, then wrap energy around them. Chi will penetrate right into the adrenals. Then take the chi about 1½ inches further down to the kidneys. In the same way that you can feel a cold blast of wind go right into your kidneys when you are cold, here feel the warmth of chi going into them.

9. Now send the chi down to the ovaries or testicles, touch the middle, and spiral (figs. 8.3, 8.4, and 8.5).

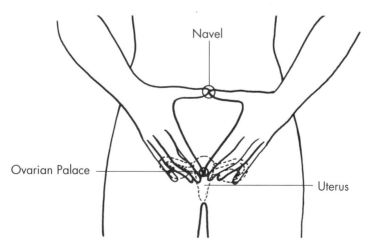

Navel

Ovarian Palace

Uterus

Fig. 8.3. Locating the Ovarian Palace

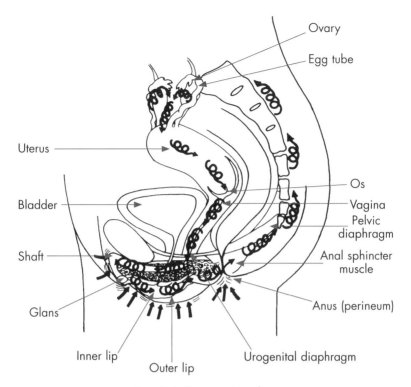

Ovary

Egg tube

Uterus

Bladder

Os

Vagina

Pelvic diaphragm

Shaft

Anal sphincter muscle

Glans

Anus (perineum)

Inner lip

Outer lip

Urogenital diaphragm

Fig. 8.4. Ovarian Breathing

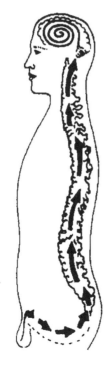

Fig. 8.5. Testicle Breathing

10. Continue down to the pubic area, to the uterus for women and to the prostate gland for men.

11. As the energy reaches the clitoris, for women, and the penis glans, for men, hold your hands near your sexual organs and feel something like a loving fire. Make it flow down to the lower tan tien, spiraling down to your sexual organs; feel the sexual energy and the loving fire.

12. As you do Testicle or Ovarian Breathing, feel the energy very gently. Men will feel it in their testicles, which will gently rise up and down, and women will feel the breath going into their ovaries.

13. Take that energy into the prostate or uterus. Hold it and feel your sexual organs transform. Put the tip of the tongue up behind the upper teeth to feel the vibrations as the sexual energy transforms.

14. Now relax into the perineum (between the sexual organs and anus), known by Taoists as the Hui Yin; feel you are relaxing down to the bottom of the sea (fig. 8.6).

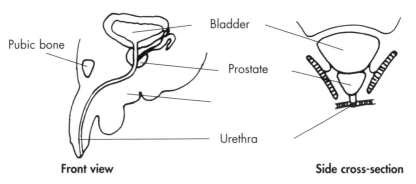

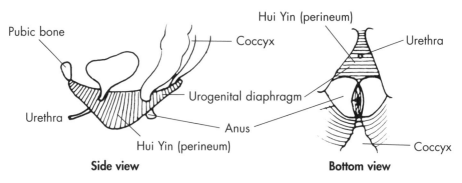

Fig. 8.6. Perineum or Hui Yin is between the sexual organ and anus.

15. Sink until you are in touch with the perineum and then it is very simple to breathe into it. Inhale, exhale; breathe into it. When you breathe into the perineum you can feel chi accumulating. Your breath is like a string pulling on the perineum.

16. Abundant energy will flow into the third eye and soon the tongue will start to vibrate; the more you relax, the more you will feel the elixir come out onto the tongue.

17. The soles of your feet will breathe in energy from the earth which flows up through the body.

Golden Elixir Chi Kung Part 2

This is an advanced internal practice Chi Kung. It circulates the ching, one of our three primary forces (the other two are chi and shen, the body force corresponding to spirit).

Ching, or "essence," our original vital energy and acquired energy, is stored in the kidneys. This practice helps to reset the body and heal the overabused digestive system.

1. Relax and breathe into your perineum; feel a ball of energy there, relax and breathe. Feel the soles of your feet breathing in earth energy, which comes up the body. Activate the sexual energy, breathe into the perineum, feel earth chi come up and combine with it. Feel that you are accumulating a chi ball.

2. Now draw up the lumbars, tuck in the sacrum, and feel the chi come up to the sacrum.

3. Let the chi spiral and accumulate in the sacrum, tilt your sacrum upward, as if you are tilting and pushing it up. Smile into the sacrum, spiral and breathe in chi. Do this a few times; when you have enough chi in your sacrum, it will start to move up.

4. Focus on the sacrum, now full of chi, as the chi goes up your spine to your skull.

5. Feel your third eye open. Touch and rub it a bit (see fig. 8.7 on page 122). Feel it open and see the light coming in, a violet light shining

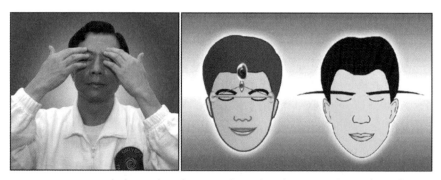

Fig. 8.7. Touch the mid-eyebrow and gently rub in a circle; smile and feel light enter; feel your eyebrows grow long.

into your brain, into your Crystal Palace. Feel your eyebrows grow out long, and gently rub them with the index and middle fingers.

6. Feel the Crystal Palace open, becoming illuminated like millions of shining crystals. As it receives light and knowledge from the universe, it reflects it to the various organs and glands (fig. 8.8), stimulating the chi in all the glands.

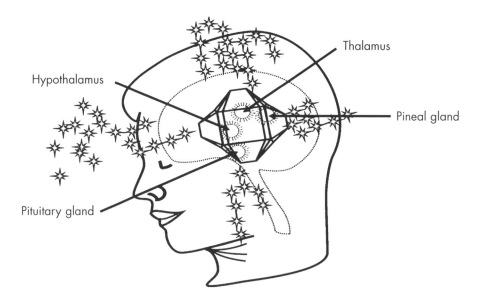

Fig. 8.8. The inside of the back of the head is called the Crystal Palace. It is also called the heavenly mirror, as it reflects light to all the glands. It can give and receive light and awaken our inner knowledge and deepest potentials.

7. Feel the energy start to move up from the sacrum to wrap around the kidneys, preparing them to produce the Golden Elixir.

8. Be aware of your heart fire; let the heart fire condense to be a loving fire, gently shining and radiating out into your lungs. The fire melts the gold metal of the lungs into a liquid that flows down to the kidneys, wrapping around them. It penetrates the kidneys softly and is absorbed into them.

9. Lightly rock on your sitting bones, while you feel fire burning in the adrenal glands on top of the kidneys further heating the kidneys. The fire wraps around the kidneys, and you can feel the force go up the body to the small brain at the back of the head.

10. Feel a very different energy arrive in the Crystal Palace. Then be aware of this energy flowing down to the mouth. The hormone system in the brain starts to activate and the fluid comes down (see fig. 8.9 on page 124).

11. At this point you will feel more saliva and the energy from the kidneys coming up and mixing with it. This is what we call the Golden Elixir, known also as the fountain of youth. All sexual energy and the energy from the glands has been activated and mixed with saliva.

12. Feel very relaxed and focus on this feeling in your mouth, and you will feel nice, cool energy and the essence of kidney ching coming in. The more you breathe and relax your mouth, the more ching will be coming.

13. The saliva increases as your third eye opens, light shines in and radiates into the glands: hypothalamus, thalamus, pineal, and pituitary.

14. Feel them activate and feel them happy and light; this is their original food.

15. The mirror on the back of your brain starts to reflect down to the thyroid and parathyroid.

16. Rock again on your sitting bones.

17. This original food, this light, beams down on your thymus gland then into the adrenal glands, kidneys, pancreas, ovaries/testicles,

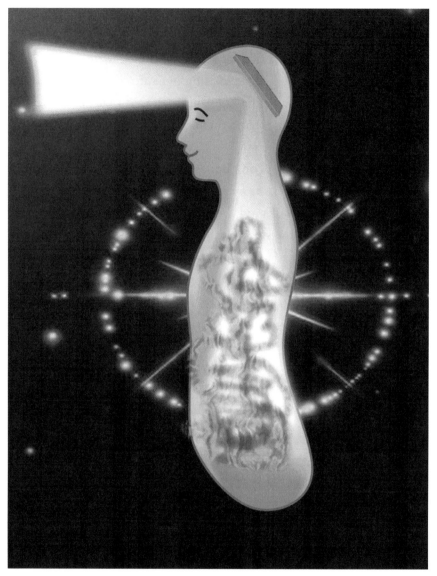

Fig. 8.9. Crystal Palace and mouth—ching fluid flows down.

and uterus/prostate. See them receiving the light as they start to recognize that "this is my original food." This is violet light, which has the lengths of all colors; it is the major food for the glands.

18. Chew the saliva, clack the teeth 36 times—in the center, left, and right sides of your mouth, then all together, 9 times each.

☯ Swallowing Golden Elixir— the Original Food

Now you are going to swallow down this elixir to the organs to increase their chi.

1. First swallow it down to the heart and lightly spiral it in the heart, to strengthen the blood circulation and blood vessels.
2. Then swallow down to the lungs, wrapping chi around them. Rub on your lungs.
3. Next swallow into the spleen: focus on the spleen to increase the shen power.
4. Then swallow down to the kidneys, increasing the ching there; rub the kidneys and feel it.
5. Finally swallow down to your liver, increasing your eye power.
6. Rest for the yin phase, the phase of stillness, of not doing anything, just being and receiving.

    The resting phase is a necessary part of the work. After the active part in meditation or Chi Kung, a yin phase allows the body to assimilate the work, to send the chi where it needs to go, and to start healing itself.
7. Then do the Crane Neck exercise 3 to 10 times (see fig. 8.10 on page 126). This improves chi circulation by activating the body's pumps: cranial, heart, lungs, and sacral. This aids all body functions, including digestion.

Golden Elixir is very important as it can increase the strength of all the organs and therefore the digestive system and all body functions. The above Chi Kung practice of swallowing down through the heart stimulates all the organs. It is a powerful exercise, involving the chi of all of the five elements: wood, fire, earth, metal, and water.

The tongue is the expression of the heart and collaborates with the orifice of the kidneys manifested in the ears. The skin is the extension

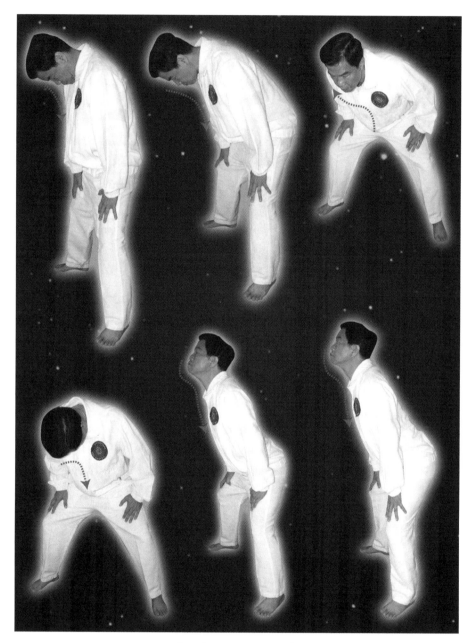

Fig. 8.10. Crane Neck

of the blood, which belongs to the heart, the fire element (fig. 8.11).

The eyes are the orifice of the liver; thus cleansing and strengthening the liver increases eye power (fig. 8.12).

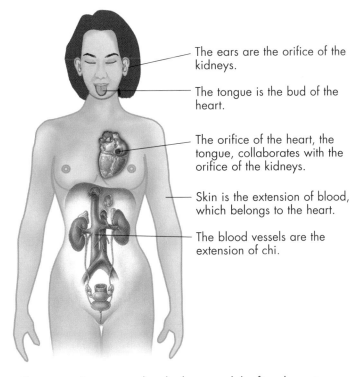

The ears are the orifice of the kidneys.

The tongue is the bud of the heart.

The orifice of the heart, the tongue, collaborates with the orifice of the kidneys.

Skin is the extension of blood, which belongs to the heart.

The blood vessels are the extension of chi.

Fig. 8.11. The tongue is connected to the heart and the fire element.

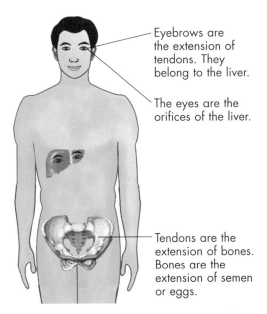

Eyebrows are the extension of tendons. They belong to the liver.

The eyes are the orifices of the liver.

Tendons are the extension of bones. Bones are the extension of semen or eggs.

Fig. 8.12. Eyes are the orifice of the liver, connected with the wood element.

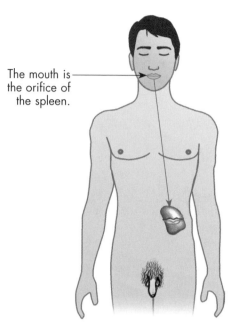

The mouth is the orifice of the spleen.

Fig. 8.13. Mouth connection to spleen and the earth element

The mouth is the orifice of the earth organs: the spleen, stomach, and pancreas (fig. 8.13).

The nose is the orifice of the lungs and large intestines, the metal organs (fig. 8.14).

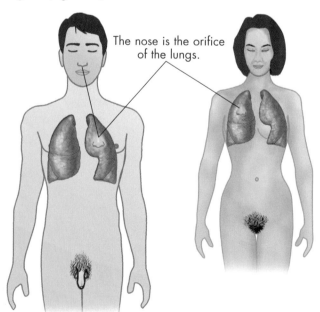

The nose is the orifice of the lungs.

Fig. 8.14. Nose is the orifice of the lungs and large intestines, the metal organs.

The ears are the orifices of the kidneys and bladder: the water organs (fig. 8.15).

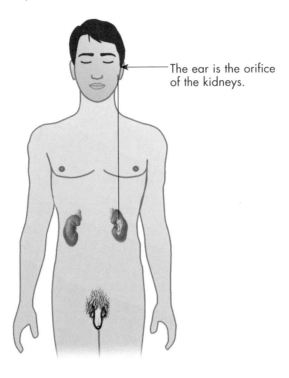

Fig. 8.15. Ears are the orifices of the kidneys and bladder, the water organs.

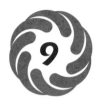

Using Pi Gu to Reset the Body's Wisdom

YOUR OWN PERSONAL BODY MAKEUP

There are many theories on types of bodies according to ayurvedic principles, blood groups, or other categories. These generally suggest that we each have a profile that defines the "type" of body we have, with its limitations or possibilities for change. A consultation with a traditional Chinese medicine practitioner, reflexologist, or acupuncturist will give you information about how Taoism might define your body. In addition, these Taoist practitioners as well as Chi Nei Tsang masseurs can rebalance your organs' energies, helping with digestion and detox processes.

Inner Alchemy Astrology can also give you some pointers. Your astrology chart will offer you insights on the quality and quantities of energy in your digestive system and also give you guidelines on your relationship with food. The calculations involved in creating each person's chart are complicated, but the work is done for you at our website: **www.universal-tao.com/InnerAlchemyAstrology**. More in-depth explanation that will guide your interpretation of your chart can be found in our book *Inner Alchemy Astrology*.

Your chart will reveal your five-element makeup, which in turn will indicate the energy strength that you have in your digestive and other organs. Your chart will also indicate current or past energy cycles that play a role in your life and health. Once you know more about the body you were born with as well as the body you have today, you will know how different foods will affect your organs.

The correspondence between the elements and organs in the body is shown in the figure below, color-coded to help you see which element energy affects which body part (fig. 9.1).

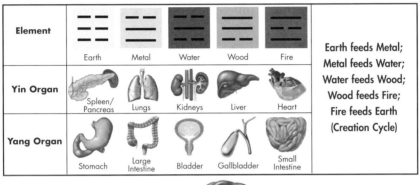

Element	Earth	Metal	Water	Wood	Fire	
Yin Organ	Spleen/ Pancreas	Lungs	Kidneys	Liver	Heart	Earth feeds Metal; Metal feeds Water; Water feeds Wood; Wood feeds Fire; Fire feeds Earth (Creation Cycle)
Yang Organ	Stomach	Large Intestine	Bladder	Gallbladder	Small Intestine	

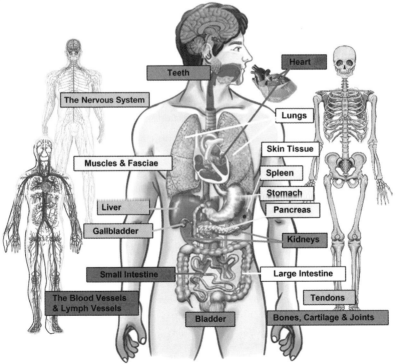

Fig. 9.1. Each of the elements is related to particular organs.

The earth element is closely related to the stomach: deficient or excessive earth will affect your stomach, pancreas, and spleen. Deficient or excessive wood element affects the liver and gallbladder; the small intestines are affected by the fire element, and the large intestine by the metal element. Five-element nutrition will show you how to boost and rebalance your fire, earth, metal, water, and wood chi.

The five-element nutrition explanations are available on the Universal Tao website:

http://www.universal-tao.com/5elements/5ElementsCDmenu.html. This web page is a wonderful interactive tool that offers you three helpful ways to access its guidance. The first tells you the foods that will help balance the elements that your Inner Alchemy Astrological chart indicates are insufficient or overly abundant. To access this information, click on the element on the diagram showing the organs, elements, and seasons. That will open the food chart, showing which foods will balance that element. The chart provides detailed information about the action of each type of food.

The second way to access the information is to choose an organ, based on your current energy or health concerns. Clicking on the organ will take you to the appropriate food chart.

The web page also offers guidance related to seasonal food choices.

RETHINKING DIET

The World Health Organization has recently cut its recommended added sugar allowance to an equivalent of twenty-five grams or six teaspoons per day. However, some popular fizzy drinks already contain the equivalent of nine teaspoons! Yogurt has an image of something healthy, yet in fact so many brands on the market contain an unhealthy amount of sugar and also a lot of questionable additives. Certain commercial yogurts have the recommended daily sugar allowance in just one portion. We are as confused as our stomachs and can no longer be sure that yogurt is a healthy choice.

For many years people have been wary of fats and particularly animal fats, to the point that margarine is often called a more healthy choice than butter, but in fact it is usually a minefield of chemicals. The cholesterol scare combined with low-fat products for dieters has seen the sugar content in commercial products go sky high. Dieters who choose low-fat products are often shooting themselves in the foot, as those products can contain high amounts of sugar, sometimes hidden under another term.

In his book *Pure White and Deadly,* nutritionist John Yudkin warned us in 1972 that sugar was a major cause of heart disease and obesity and that refining it and removing nutrients that are good for us makes matters worse. Yet here we are today consuming it under many hidden names. "Light" drinks, with no sugar, are usually very sweet tasting, due to the high level of aspartame or other doubtful sugar substitutes. In fact it has been shown that these chemicals have a similar effect on the body's insulin levels as actual sugar. So one more poison has been added to our shopping basket. These products are so sweet that they help to keep the "sweet tooth" as needy as possible, rather than weaning the mouth away from such cravings.

If you are buying processed foods, then it is up to you as the consumer, or parent of the consumer, to do your own research into what you should and should not eat. If you rely on convenience foods, then reading the lists of ingredients on the packet is essential, but not easy, despite the constant battle of consumer groups to introduce more clarity. Often the font in which the lists are written is very small and difficult to read (see fig. 9.2 on page 134).

Buying simple, fresh, preferably organic foods and preparing them yourself is a good solution; if that is not possible, be more aware of what you are buying to eat. Rethinking what you eat is essential to resetting your body system. We have recommended reading on this at the end of this book.

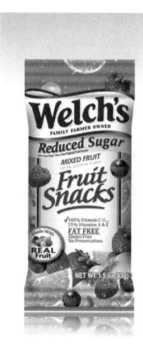

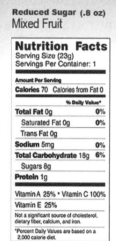

Fig. 9.2. Can you actually read these ingredients?

Food Poverty

The U.S. Government Supplementary Nutrition Assistance Program (formerly known as food stamps) serves 48 million people who are "food insecure," that is, too poor to buy enough food. Convenience foods are often cheaper than fresh ingredients for home cooking, and in poorer districts, grocers close down while fast food outlets flourish. Many of the food poor are classed as overweight, as the cheapest convenience foods can be the worst ones for our bodies. At such a level of poverty, buying fresh fruits and vegetables is not affordable. The real cost of fruits and vegetables has risen by 24 percent since the 1980s while the cost of sodas has dropped by 27 percent.

The U.S. Government massively subsidizes corn, much of which ends up in the "junk food" industry, particularly as high fructose corn syrup, yet relatively little subsidy goes to fruits and vegetables.

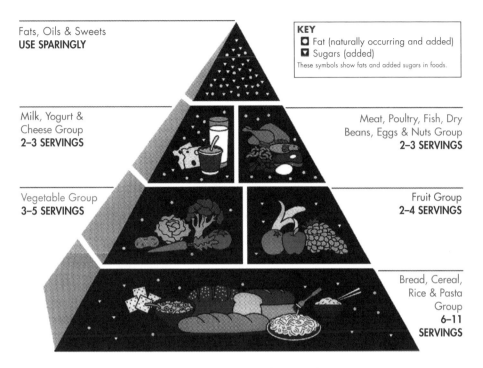

Fig. 9.3. USDA Food Pyramid

Grains and the Modern Diet

Throughout our lives, starting when we are babies, grains are a major part of our diet: we have pasta, spaghetti, cereals, noodles, bread, or breakfast cereals every day (fig. 9.3). A Western meal is often 60 to 80 percent grain.

Some people live on sandwiches; they are easy to buy and easy to prepare. We find very clean kitchens in many Western homes, as not much food preparation is taking place. In a traditional Chinese kitchen there is a lot more activity and the preparation and cooking of food often makes the kitchen dirtier or messier, but the Chinese use fewer grains.

However, many people are now being diagnosed as wheat or gluten intolerant or even allergic. After a certain amount of such food in the system, the body needs to detoxify. In these cases, we have discovered that if you stop eating wheat or gluten for a while and wait, the body is quite likely to reset itself and accept it again afterward. Chi and good chewing will also help the body to reset and accept the food again. After following the Pi Gu program described in this book, the body will start to tell you what it needs and will recover from its state of confusion, which causes it to express intolerance to various foods.

Getting to Know the Good Grains

Not only do we consume a lot of grains, but most of them are missing the germ and husk, which contain essential vitamins and nutrients. Today we consume a lot of bleached flour and white rice. In fact the germ and husk are sold back to us in health food supplements. Traditionally in Thailand, the rich ate white, refined rice and got fat, and the farmers ate red rice, or "horse rice" as it was called. In fact, prisoners were fed on red rice too, so today in Thailand we say that you look like a jailbird if you eat red rice, although many people are now doing it, having understood that it is better for health.

"Live" foods, that is, foods that can be germinated, have vitality that "dead" foods do not. In the Tao Garden kitchens we use five different varieties of rice, all of which can be germinated. We soak them for one day and in the morning we look to see if they have germinated. If they have started to sprout, that means that the rice still has life, and we will cook it; other rices will only ferment after a long time, as they have lost their vitality.

Fruit

Fruit contains many valuable nutrients as well as fiber. But its sugar content—as fructose—is also high. Eating fruit provides nutrients, fiber, and chewing exercise. Drinking fruit juice, however, does not provide the full fiber content and it does not need chewing, so not much saliva is produced to aid digestion. The sugar content of fruit juice can be very high: it is easy to drink but has a dramatic effect on blood sugar level. This is part of the diabetes problem today. Some fruit juices or "fruit drinks" are worse than others, as there are added sugars and preserving or coloring chemicals in them.

BEGINNING PI GU AT HOME

As a first step, if you do not want to commit to advanced darkroom meditations, you can change the way you chew your food, as we have described in chapter 4. In this way you could change the way you eat every day.

Then try Pi Gu one day a week. On that day, just cut down on food and eat peanuts, walnuts, red prunes, dates, or goji berries. Chew them well. After that, have an apple or pear. Then start practicing the simplest Chi Kung in this book. If you try Pi Gu once a week, you will be giving your body a rest from grains and breaking the cycle you have had since babyhood, but you will not be totally halting your digestive system with all the problems that can bring.

Doing Pi Gu even once a week will not only be good for you but you will eat less. If you spend the right time chewing you will have to eat less, easily 10 to 50 percent less. But you will not get hunger pangs, as you will have so much saliva and chi inside of you.

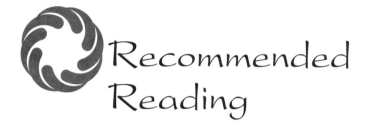

Recommended Reading

FOR CHI KUNG AND MEDITATIONS

All of Mantak Chia's books on the Universal Healing Tao practices are based on the Taoist view of the universe. After having read this book on the practice of Pi Gu Chi Kung, you might particularly like to read or reread the following books by Mantak Chia:

Basic Practices of the Universal Healing Tao: An Illustrated Guide to Levels 1 through 6 with coauthor William U. Wei. Rochester, Vt.: Destiny Books, 2013.

Craniosacral Chi Kung with coauthor Joyce Thom. Rochester, Vt.: Destiny Books, 2016.

Golden Elixir Chi Kung. Rochester, Vt.: Destiny Books, 2005.

Healing Light of the Tao: Foundational Practices to Awaken Chi Energy. Rochester, Vt.: Destiny Books, 2008.

Healing Love through the Tao: Cultivating Female Sexual Energy. Rochester, Vt.: Destiny Books, 2005.

The Inner Smile: Increasing Chi through the Cultivation of Joy. Rochester, Vt.: Destiny Books, 2008.

Tan Tien Chi Kung. Rochester, Vt.: Destiny Books, 2004.

Taoist Secrets of Love: Cultivating Male Sexual Energy with coauthor Michael Winn. Santa Fe, N.M.: Aurora Press, 1984.

DETOXIFICATION

The following books by Mantak Chia will be especially helpful regarding gaining more understanding of the need for and ways to detoxify the body:

Chi Nei Tsang: Chi Massage for the Vital Organs. Rochester, Vt.: Destiny Books, 2007; and *Advanced Chi Nei Tsang: Enhancing Chi Energy in the Vital Organs.* Rochester, Vt.: Destiny Books, 2009.

Chi Self Massage: The Taoist Way of Rejuvenation. Rochester, Vt.: Destiny Books, 2006.

Cosmic Detox: A Taoist Approach to Internal Cleansing with coauthor William U. Wei. Rochester, Vt.: Destiny Books, 2011.

The Six Healing Sounds: Taoist Techniques for Balancing Chi. Rochester, Vt.: Destiny Books, 2009.

INTERPRETING YOUR OWN BODY

As mentioned in the text, an invaluable resource for deeper understanding of Chinese astrology and your own five-element makeup is the following book by Mantak Chia and Christine Harkness-Giles:

Inner Alchemy Astrology: Practical Techniques for Controlling Your Destiny. Rochester, Vt.: Destiny Books, 2013.

FOR DIET

To further explore the dietary suggestions in this book you may want to read the books below by Mantak Chia and other authors:

Cosmic Nutrition by Mantak Chia and William U. Wei. Rochester, Vt.: Destiny Books, 2012.

The Diet Myth: The Real Science Behind What We Eat by Tim Spector. London: Weidenfeld & Nicolson, 2015.

Fat Chance—the Bitter Truth about Sugar by Dr. Robert Lustig. London: Penguin, 2013.

Fats that Heal and Fats that Kill by Udo Erasmus. Summertown, Tenn.: Book Publishing Company, 1993.

The Great Cholesterol Myth by Jonny Bowden and Stephen Sinatra. Vancouver, Canada: Fair Winds Press, 2012.

Pure White and Deadly by John Yudkin. London: Davis-Poynter, 1972. (As well as his other books on nutrition.)

The Sugar Fix by Richard Johnson and Timothy Gower. New York: Simon and Schuster, 2009.

The Tao of Balanced Diet by Dr. Stephen T. Chang. Reno, Nev.: Tao Longevity, 1987.

The Tao of the Delicious by Mantak Chia and Shashi Solluna. (This book is available through the Tao Garden bookshop. E-mail Tao Garden for more information at info@tao-garden.com.)

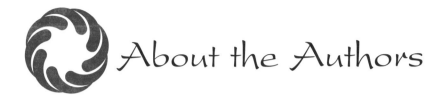

About the Authors

MANTAK CHIA

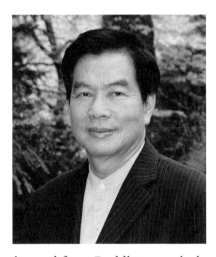

Mantak Chia has been studying the Taoist approach to life since childhood. His mastery of this ancient knowledge, enhanced by his study of other disciplines, has resulted in the development of the Universal Healing Tao system, which is now being taught throughout the world.

Mantak Chia was born in Thailand to Chinese parents in 1944. When he was six years old, he learned from Buddhist monks how to sit and "still the mind." While in grammar school he learned traditional Thai boxing, and he soon went on to acquire considerable skill in aikido, yoga, and Tai Chi. His studies of the Taoist way of life began in earnest when he was a student in Hong Kong, ultimately leading to his mastery of a wide variety of esoteric disciplines, with the guidance of several masters, including Master I Yun, Master Meugi, Master Cheng Yao Lun, and Master Pan Yu. To better understand the mechanisms behind healing energy, he also studied Western anatomy and medical sciences.

Master Chia has taught his system of healing and energizing practices to tens of thousands of students and trained more than two thousand instructors and practitioners throughout the world. He has established centers for Taoist study and training in many countries around the globe. In 1990 and in 2012, he was honored by the International Congress of Chinese Medicine and Qi Gong (Chi Kung), which named him the Qi Gong Master of the Year.

CHRISTINE HARKNESS-GILES

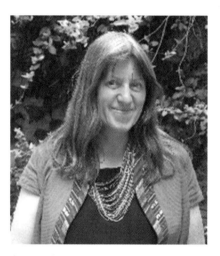

Christine is a certified instructor in the Universal Healing Tao system, and a feng shui consultant and teacher, born in the UK and presently living in London. She has been a student of Taoism for many years, studying feng shui, Chinese astrology, the I Ching and other traditional Taoist arts, notably with Master Joseph Yu, founder of the Feng Shui Research Centre (FSRC), as well as promoting and teaching the Taoist arts in Europe.

Meeting Mantak Chia and learning the Universal Healing Tao practices provided the "missing link" for her between Taoist knowledge and living Taoist philosophy in today's world. She has studied and practiced Pi Gu with Master Chia during the darkroom retreats and in workshops in Europe.

Christine teaches Mantak Chia's particular form of traditional Chinese astrology—Inner Alchemy Astrology. It reveals people's five-element makeup, making it easier for them to understand Chi Kung and meditation techniques to balance and enhance their own Original Chi and their changing energy cycles. She also regularly uses Inner Alchemy Astrology with her students and feng shui clients, teaching the method at home in the Eurostar triangle of London, Paris, and Brussels, as well as in other parts of the world, including Hawaii.

The Universal Healing Tao System and Training Center

THE UNIVERSAL HEALING TAO SYSTEM

The ultimate goal of Taoist practice is to transcend physical boundaries through the development of the soul and the spirit within the human. That is also the guiding principle behind the Universal Healing Tao, a practical system of self-development that enables individuals to complete the harmonious evolution of their physical, mental, and spiritual bodies. Through a series of ancient Chinese meditative and internal energy exercises, the practitioner learns to increase physical energy, release tension, improve health, practice self-defense, and gain the ability to heal him- or herself and others. In the process of creating a solid foundation of health and well-being in the physical body, the practitioner also creates the basis for developing his or her spiritual potential by learning to tap into the natural energies of the sun, moon, earth, stars, and other environmental forces.

The Universal Healing Tao practices are derived from ancient techniques rooted in the processes of nature. They have been gathered and integrated into a coherent, accessible system for well-being that works directly with the life force, or chi, that flows through the meridian system of the body.

Master Chia has spent years developing and perfecting techniques for teaching these traditional practices to students around the world through ongoing classes, workshops, private instruction, and healing sessions, as well as books, video, audio products, YouTube demonstrations, and online classes. Go to www.universal-tao.com for more information.

THE UNIVERSAL HEALING TAO TRAINING CENTER

The Tao Garden Resort and Training Center in northern Thailand is the home of Master Chia and serves as the worldwide headquarters for Universal Healing Tao activities. This integrated wellness, holistic health, and training center is situated on eighty acres surrounded by the beautiful Himalayan foothills near the historic walled city of Chiang Mai. The serene setting includes flower and herb gardens ideal for meditation, open-air pavilions for practicing Chi Kung, and a health and fitness spa.

The center offers classes year round, as well as summer and winter retreats. It can accommodate two hundred students, and group leasing can be arranged. For information on courses, books, products, and other Universal Healing Tao resources, see below.

RESOURCES

Universal Healing Tao Center
274 Moo 7, Luang Nua, Doi Saket, Chiang Mai, 50220 Thailand
Tel: (66)(53) 495-596 Fax: (66)(53) 495-852
E-mail: universaltao@universal-tao.com
Web site: www.universal-tao.com

For information on retreats and the health spa, contact:
Tao Garden Health Spa & Resort
E-mail: info@tao-garden.com, taogarden@hotmail.com
Web site: www.tao-garden.com

Good Chi • Good Heart • Good Intention

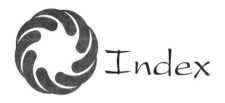

Index

Page numbers in *italics* indicate illustrations.